Your Heart House

An Artisan's Approach™ to Understanding Heart Health

AARUSH MANCHANDA, M.D., FACC, FASNC

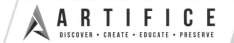

ARTIFICE
DISCOVER • CREATE • EDUCATE • PRESERVE

DISCOVER challenges,
CREATE solutions, EDUCATE people,
and PRESERVE lives

For my Biji

Contents

"Biji has passed," said my uncle, with tears in his eyes.

I looked up at him in disbelief, a gigantic lump forming in my throat. I couldn't fathom the idea of never seeing my beloved grandmother again.

It was at that moment that I decided I wanted to be a heart surgeon. I was 15 years old.

About the Author

Aarush Manchanda is in the trenches of heart disease every day—and has been for 12 years. After receiving his medical degree from the Maulana Azad Medical College at the University of Delhi, India, he immigrated to the United States where he completed his internship and residency.

Dr. Manchanda is board certified in five specialties: internal medicine, cardiovascular disease, nuclear cardiology, cardiac computed tomography, and echocardiography. He currently works as a staff cardiologist at Cedar City Heart Clinic and as the Medical Director of Cardiovascular Services at Cedar City Hospital in Cedar City, Utah. In this role, he's brought multimodality cardiology imaging, once thought to be only a fantasy for the rural community of Cedar City, into the realm of everyday practice.

He has earned many top awards as a student, resident, and researcher, including the Resident of the Year Award from George Washington University and the Veterans Affairs Hospital in Washington D.C., and the Best Resident Research Award from Geisinger Medical Center in Danville, Pennsylvania. He has continued to be a leader in the medical community by educating others and taking on residents as a chief fellow at Geisinger Medical Center in Danville, Pennsylvania.

Dr. Manchanda has made it his life's work to facilitate a health-conscious community. His genuine concern for the health of his patients is a testament to his dedication and his balanced approach to patient relations. To develop individualized plans for healthy lifestyle changes, he continuously seeks ways to make understanding complex health issues accessible to everyone. Dr. Manchanda creates a trusting and personal relationship with each patient, and understands that the most successful approach to health care is one that takes into account the overall wellbeing of a patient.

Dr. Manchanda lives with his wife and daughter in Cedar City, Utah and spends his leisure time skiing, playing golf, and meditating.

PART 1

Introduction

A Note to My Readers

Heart disease is the number one cause of death in the United States—and the world. Every 40 seconds, one American dies from cardiovascular disease, which claims more lives than all forms of cancer combined.[1]

Heart disease is an umbrella term for a range of conditions affecting your heart. It's my observation that most people—whether they have heart disease or not—don't understand the basics of the heart, and the importance of their heart health. They don't know the difference between a heart attack, cardiac arrest, and heart failure. And, they don't understand how conditions that affect one part of the heart—for example, the arteries—can negatively impact other parts of the heart, such as the walls. I've been practicing cardiology and related medicine for 12 years, and have witnessed how this lack of understanding leads not only to fear and hopelessness for patients and their families, but also to poorer patient health.

That's why I wrote this book: My goal is to empower patients through knowledge. I believe knowledge is the first step toward changing behavior.

For many people, a heart attack is the first sign of heart disease. And while most people live through their first heart attack, about 23% of women and 18% of men die within the year.[2] Those who do live longer live with a damaged heart muscle. In my practice, I've seen how educating patients and getting them involved in their care can help improve their health and even save lives. Patients who clearly understand their conditions and treatments are often more motivated to engage in their heart health and adhere to prescribed treatments.

Most of the major risk factors for heart disease—hypertension, diet, lack of physical activity, smoking, and obesity—are related to lifestyle choices.

Each of us must be involved in our care to combat heart disease; and, we have to understand how our heart works and what we need to do to stay healthy.

If you're at risk for heart disease, it's especially essential that you know how your heart works and what can go wrong. If you have a heart condition, you need to understand the problem and how doctors will treat it. Doing so will help you stick with your treatment plan, be less suspicious of suggestions your doctor makes, and better be able to make healthy choices that can significantly impact your health and survival.

The landscape of medicine is changing dramatically; patients are no longer willing to simply accept "doctor's orders" and are rightfully demanding more say in their treatment. But to be involved in making decisions regarding your treatment, you must first understand the structure and function of the heart. Then, you'll be able to make informed choices about your health and well-being.

My goal is to shed light on the mystery. I'm going to show you that the heart is fundamentally a pump, complete with plumbing and electrical systems, so you can begin to grasp what's going on inside your body. Honestly, it's as straightforward as the systems that power your home. The information in this book is relevant to every human being. I hope you will take the time to read it and use what you learn to live a healthier and more rewarding life. Your heart will thank you for it!

—Aarush Manchanda, M.D., FACC, FASNC
Cedar City, Utah, 2016

How to Use This Book

Through *Your Heart House,* you'll be able to equip yourself with knowledge about your heart, its potential problems and treatment options. Each part of your heart has its own section in this book, and each of those sections is presented the same way. Let's use the valves section as an example: First I help you to understand what the heart's valves are and how they work; next, I explain the problems that can arise and the symptoms of these issues, followed by their causes. Then I describe how we diagnose these problems, and finally how we treat them.

Sections 3-8 conclude with a lifestyle chapter: my recommendations as to how you can take the best care of that particular part of your heart. At the end of each of these lifestyle chapters, I provide you with practical tips. I've also included Artisan Reviews, brief summaries that provide you with the chapter's key concepts, at the end of many of the chapters. Also, throughout the book, you'll find some interesting—and sometimes surprising—facts from the world of cardiology. You'll recognize these bonuses throughout the book by their icons:

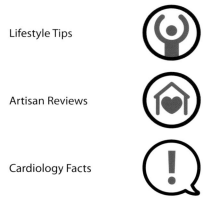

Lifestyle Tips

Artisan Reviews

Cardiology Facts

You'll also notice quotes from me throughout the book. Every one of these quotes is a piece of information or advice that I give to my patients. You'll recognize them because they'll look like this:

There's a wealth of medical information on the Internet: Facebook feeds, Dr. Google's advice, hundreds of thousands of medical publications—and more. Don't get overwhelmed. Trust your instinct and seek out reliable, expert sources.

While the book stays true to my Heart House Analogy—which I'll explain soon—I've also included medical terms so you can readily understand how the concepts that I teach relate to what you may be hearing from your doctor. There's a glossary of medical terms and an index in the back of the book, but you don't have to memorize any of these technical words. Throughout this book, I'll help you understand the parts and functions of your heart in the simplest of terms.

Your Heart House can be read cover to cover, but it's also designed as a reference tool for patients. If, for example, your doctor has said you have a problem with your heart's walls or one of its valves, you can turn to the sections that cover those parts of your heart to better understand your condition and what will likely be done to address it. Essentially, you can become a novice cardiologist so you can participate in your care.

Finding My Passion

You might say that my career as a cardiologist began when I was about 8 years old.

My family—my father, mother, sister, me, and my Biji (the Punjabi word for mom or grandmother)—lived in a comfortable three-bedroom home in Delhi, India, where I was born in 1980. Both of my parents were physicians, but that wasn't the primary reason I was so interested in medicine, and especially in heart health. You see, my first heart patient was Biji.

When I was 8 and my sister was 5, our grandmother had her first heart attack. Until then she had been the primary adult caretaker in our lives, cooking and caring for us so that my parents could tend to their busy clinical practices. Biji came home from the hospital with a sack of pills and instructions to rest, and to avoid both stress and too many stairs. Although Delhi was a city of nearly seven million people, there were no established heart surgery facilities. The nearest was a plane ride away.

After her heart attack, my parents had me sleep in Biji's bed with her. That way if she woke up in distress or needed something, I would be there to help or summon my parents. My Biji was much beloved in the family, as a doting grandmother and mom. The heart attack was upsetting, especially because the same event had taken my grandfather's life not long before. He'd complained of shortness of breath late one night, so my dad and uncle called for a taxi to take him to the hospital. On the way, the driver had to brake suddenly to avoid a collision, and everyone was pitched violently forward. My grandfather died in my father's arms in the back seat of a cab.

Biji was less active than she had been before the heart attack, but nearly every evening she'd get dressed and sit out on the veranda where we kids would play. Vendors roamed the streets selling fruit, sweets, nuts, roasted corn, and ice cream. She'd give us each a couple of rupees to buy a treat.

Sometimes at night she'd wake up with an attack of angina (chest pain), short of breath, sweaty, and rubbing the left side of her chest and her left arm. I'd fetch her bag of medicines, and she'd tell me to give her one or two of these tiny pills—Sorbitrate—that she placed under her tongue. Sorbitrate (isosorbide dinitrate) dilates the blood vessels, facilitating better circulation and alleviating some strain from the heart muscle. After that, she would sleep and wake up feeling well. Later, an uncle who was a cardiologist in the United States came to visit and brought her nitroglycerin in spray form. "That American stuff really works," she told me.

From the beginning of these episodes, Biji swore me to secrecy. When the first bit of daylight brightened the window, my grandmother would insist I not tell anyone about her pain the previous night. "You mustn't worry your mother and father about it," she'd instruct adamantly. "I don't want to end up in the hospital and cause a lot of trouble. I've caused enough as it is."

In spite of her condition, Biji soldiered on, year after year. One day when I was in 10th grade, sitting in my classroom, I looked out the window and saw one of my uncles approaching. He summoned me outside and told me that Biji had suffered a fatal heart attack. It was my first experience with death and grief. I felt as though I'd lost a mother. The entire family was emotionally devastated. She had died at nine o'clock in the morning. By the time the ambulance arrived at our home with her body, rigor mortis had set it in. We struggled to get her in the house where the traditional washing and preparation for cremation took place. My father rarely shed a tear when he was sad. This day he—all of us—sobbed uncontrollably.

At that point in my education, I was expected to begin making choices that would define my professional life. Biji's death confirmed my desire to be a doctor. I told my friends, "I'm going to be a heart surgeon."

My first surgery rotation cured me of that ambition. The patient had bladder cancer, and my job was to hold a retractor—a clamp—all day. The surgery lasted more than 10 hours, and the patient died a day or so later. Not for me, I realized. I wanted to help people before they needed surgery.

In university, few other people felt the pull toward cardiology that I had. Many of my classmates dropped out or switched majors for specialties that were less challenging or more mainstream. I've always gotten a thrill out of learning things that few other people know. It provides me with the opportunity to think outside of the box and find new creative ways to treat those who are suffering.

After graduating from the Maulana Azad Medical College at the University of Delhi, I continued my education in the United States, ultimately receiving five board certifications. In 2009, as I was deciding where I would settle in the U.S., President Obama mentioned Geisinger Medical Center and Utah's Intermountain Health Care system as examples of the nation's best and most efficient institutions. It happened that Intermountain was looking for someone to head a new cardiology program and to build it from scratch. One thing led to another, and that's where I ended up, as Medical Director of Cardiovascular Services at Cedar City Hospital in Cedar City, Utah.

At Cedar City, I've had the opportunity to create a cardiology program from the ground up, hiring and training staff and implementing the latest in best practices. I've used this facility as my opportunity to create a health-conscious community. I've always believed that an informed population is a healthier population, so I've always strived to make complicated and often confusing medical concepts easier for patients to understand.

From the start, I wanted to go beyond what the medical profession is doing today: focusing on treating established disease with procedures and surgeries at the expense of education and prevention. It's not enough to simply focus on fixing patients and sending them on their way.

I try to maintain a relationship with my patients throughout their care, checking in with them every six months to a year. After several years of caring for a wide variety of individuals and spending time explaining their hearts and conditions to them, I decided it was time to write a book to provide my patients with support in between check-ins. And, I wanted to help a much wider audience better understand their bodies and their health. My objective is to empower my readers with the knowledge they need to make intelligent, informed decisions in cooperation with their health care teams, and to equip them with the means to improve their heart health.

If my grandma were alive today, I'm certain she'd be very proud of me! After all, her "little doctor," who kept her secret stories in his heart, has become a scientific, highly educated cardiologist with an Artisan's Approach™.

The Artisan's Approach™

Long before health care was a science, it was a craft. And, millennia before doctors were scientists, they were artisans. Even Hippocrates, who's often considered the father of medicine, referred to medicine as an art, and it's only in recent decades that doctors have relied primarily on research and formulas to guide them in diagnosing and treating patients.

While science has provided a wealth of tools for physicians to use, I believe we still need to view and practice medicine as an art, for it is, indeed, both a science and an art. Patients aren't just a set of symptoms in a study, and caring for them involves more than following one-size-fits-all instructions. I consider myself an artisan. That's why, as a cardiologist, I've developed the Artisan's Approach™: a means of treating and empowering patients while recognizing each patient's individuality and specific heart issues.

Artisans work at their craft by hand. There's a personal touch to their creations, and no two are exactly alike. Similarly, no two patients are the same, and as an artisan, I'm not content to follow a cookie-cutter treatment plan. Rather, I think outside the box, looking for ways to effectively address patients' heart health and involve them in their own care.

Most people know that the heart is one of the most complex organs in the body, but they might be shocked to learn exactly how this multifaceted marvel works. As an artisan, I have the ability to dissect complex information and share it in a way that makes it easier to comprehend. Using my Artisan's Approach™, I've created an analogy, called the Heart House, to help you understand this incredible organ in your body. This analogy is essentially a new language, which can be adopted by both cardiologists and patients alike, to help resolve the disconnect patients often feel with their heart doctors. Hopefully, my explanation will be easier to comprehend than most medical textbooks.

PART 2

Your Heart House: The Basics

CHAPTER 1

More Than Spectators

An Anxious Subject

Sitting across from me is Robert. He's in his mid-40s and is perspiring lightly. I imagine if I were to take his pulse, it would be racing. These telltale signs of stress are common when patients listen to their diagnosis and prognosis from a cardiologist, delivered in what must sound like a foreign language. In some respects, it is a foreign language, saved only for doctors and medical personnel.

Like most of my patients, Robert has never thought much about the health of his heart, despite the fact that it's a crucial organ responsible for pumping oxygen and nutrient-rich blood to every other part of his body, including his brain. Most of us just assume—or hope—our hearts will do their jobs and work well for as long as needed. Well, now Robert is having shooting pain running through his upper chest—the kind of pain that's hard to ignore and so often serves as a wake-up call that you do indeed have a heart and right now it might not be functioning as it should.

Thankfully, Robert's family had hurried him to the hospital (as all families should do when someone is experiencing unexplained chest pain), where he underwent a battery of tests. Now he's sitting in my office fearful and sweating. The doctor in the emergency department has already told Robert he didn't have a heart attack, and now he's waiting anxiously to understand what has happened to him.

As I start to explain his condition, Robert fidgets and looks at the certificates on the wall. I can see that he's starting to tune me out. It's at moments like these that I realize how many of my patients view their hearts as disengaged, casual spectators, removed from the situation. Heart health scares them and they feel they have little control over it, so they prefer to assume that doctors like me will fix it if something goes wrong. Often, even after they've had a good scare (chest pain being a common one), many patients feel that it's all just too confusing and complex, and fail to actively engage in caring for their hearts.

Cardiology, like many other areas of medicine, can understandably be overwhelming. For most patients, a heart attack is unexpected. Many don't understand even the basics of what has happened. But, the heart is much easier to understand than many realize. Each part has a specific function; all the parts work together to allow you to do the activities you enjoy each day.

For several years I've used the analogy of a house for the heart. As an artisan, I created this comparison to help my patients easily grasp how the cardiac system works and what happens when things go awry. My Heart House

Your Heart House

Aorta = Driveway

Plumbing = Coronary Arteries
Chambers = Rooms

Valves = Doors

Electrical System = Rhythm

Myocardium = Walls

Pericardium = Siding

analogy draws direct comparisons between parts of a house—their functions and potential issues—to parts of the heart. This analogy may seem strange at first, but your heart has the same parts as your house—rooms, plumbing, walls, electricity, doors, siding, and a driveway—and functions in much the same way.

I've found that making these comparisons helps patients remember the details relevant to them and their specific conditions. More importantly, once they understand what's happening in their hearts, they can join me in determining the best course of action to keep them healthy and well, or the best way to restore their health. In the next chapter, we'll take a look at my Heart House analogy.

CHAPTER 2

Your Heart House

Your heart is a pump: a muscular organ, about the size of your fist, located in the middle of your chest, slightly to the left of your breastbone. A man's heart typically weighs about 10 ounces and a woman's heart weighs about eight ounces. This amazing organ pumps approximately 2,000 gallons of blood through your body every single day! Together, your heart and blood vessels comprise your *cardiovascular system*, which circulates blood and oxygen around your body.

To best understand the individual parts of the heart, you need a general sense of the anatomy of the heart as a whole. The heart has a top floor and a bottom floor, a right side and a left side. So, think of your heart as a two-story duplex with two rooms on each floor.

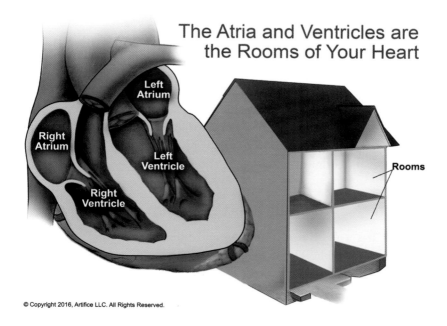

The Atria and Ventricles are the Rooms of Your Heart

The two rooms on the top floor of your heart are called the *right atrium* and the *left atrium*. Similarly, the two rooms on the bottom floor of your heart are called the *right ventricle* and the *left ventricle*. These are the four chambers, or rooms, of your heart. They work together to enable your heart to fulfill its purpose: pumping to ensure that blood flows throughout your body.

The Right Side of Your Heart

When you see colored drawings of the heart, the right side is generally shown on the left side of the picture, as if you're looking at someone else's heart rather than at your own in a mirror. The right side is also usually depicted in blue. That's because the blood in the right side of your heart has just returned to the heart from the rest of the body, which has used the oxygen and nutrients in the blood. It's colored in blue to demonstrate that it lacks oxygen. The oxygen-depleted blood enters the heart through two large veins (the *inferior* and *superior vena cava*), emptying into the *right atrium,* the top room of the right side of the heart. As the atrium contracts, the blood flows down through the *tricuspid valve* to the right ventricle, or bottom floor, and then out the *pulmonary artery* to the lungs, where it picks up oxygen from the air in the lungs. Think of your lungs as the air filter—they clean the blood by removing carbon dioxide and exchanging it for oxygen.

The Left Side of Your Heart

Once your blood has obtained oxygen in the lungs, it flows back into the left side of your heart through the *pulmonary veins,* once again starting at the top floor, in the left atrium, and then flowing down through the *mitral valve* into the left ventricle. From there, the left ventricle gives a large contraction and the blood is expelled from the heart or, in the Heart House analogy, it goes out the driveway (the *aorta*), flowing to the rest of the body. This cycle is vital to the proper functioning of your entire body.

Your Heart's Rhythm

Your heart has a rhythm of pumping and filling that keeps blood flowing throughout your body. Think about a baby's bath toy that's meant to fill up with water. First, you must squeeze the toy; then, when it's underwater, you release it to let it fill. The same thing takes places when your heart beats. It first pumps blood out through the arteries; this phase of the heartbeat is called *systole.* Then it rests, known as *diastole*, to refill the rooms of the heart. Your heart beats in this natural cycle as it pumps blood out to the two circuits: the lung circuit and the body circuit. A man's average heart rate is about 70 beats per minute. Since a woman's heart is typically smaller than a man's, her heart beats a bit faster, usually around 78 beats per minute.

The plumbing in your house moves water from room to room. Similarly, your arteries transport blood. Electricity provides power to your house in the same way the electrical system of your heart keeps the heart powered up and pumping. The walls of your house provide structure just like the *myocardium* (your heart's walls) does for your heart. The siding provides some extra protection to the walls in your house; we call this the *pericardium* in the heart. The driveway is the main exit out of your house; it's like the aorta, a large artery that allows blood to exit to the rest of your body.

Heart Problems

Heart problems always occur in one of six parts of your Heart House:

The Parts of Your Heart House	Common Problems
Plumbing (Arteries and Veins)	Coronary Artery Disease (CAD)
Walls (Myocardium)	Heart Failure
Electricity (Heartbeat/Rhythm)	Arrhythmias, palpitations
Doors (Valves)	Valvular Heart Disease
Siding (Pericardium)	Pericarditis
Driveway (Aorta)	Aortic aneurysm, rupture, dissection

We'll discuss all of these issues in the coming chapters. Meanwhile, please understand that while certain areas of your house can work independently of each other (for instance, the plumbing works regardless of the condition of the roof, and the electrical system functions without the doors), in truth your house is all one large system that depends on the performance of each part. Each element combined with the others strengthens the overall structure and contributes key components that provide stability and functionality. Without walls, the plumbing and electrical systems would be exposed. Without the driveway, nothing could come in and out of the house. The same applies to the different parts of your heart. While they can get sick, damaged, or diseased in isolation, this is the exception rather than the rule. Most of the time, when one system fails, other systems are affected. Achieving and maintaining heart health affects each of the systems in your body.

The heart's job is to get oxygenated blood out to your whole body, then back again to refill the blood with more oxygen. There are two circuits: the lung circuit and the body circuit. In both circuits, the blood enters at the top and moves to the bottom of your heart before being sent to the lungs or the body. The blood on the right side comes in from the body and goes out to the lungs; the blood on the left comes in from the lungs and goes out to the body. The plumbing, electricity, walls, driveway, and siding of your heart all work together to make this happen.

CHAPTER 3

Causes of Heart Problems

The "Big Two" causes of heart disease are *diabetes* (elevated glucose in the blood caused by an inability to produce sufficient insulin) and *hypertension* (high blood pressure). However, there are additional risk factors that increase your chance of heart disease, and they fall into two broad categories: acquired and congenital. An *acquired risk factor* is one you develop over your lifetime; *congenital risk factors* are those you were born with. In this section, we'll focus mainly on acquired risk factors, which can be divided into two subcategories: modifiable and non-modifiable.

Non-Modifiable Risk Factors

Let's first talk about the risk factors that are beyond your control: the non-modifiable risk factors. You may be asking, "If I can't do anything about these risk factors, then what's the point of discussing them?" The answer is simple: If you know about these risk factors, you can take extra precautions in the areas that you can affect.

Non-modifiable risk factors include age, gender, race, and family history. The older you are, the more likely you are to suffer from heart disease. Just like your house, when the materials of your heart start aging, they may not work as well anymore. And while our bodies aren't as simple as our houses (we can't just swap in new parts like we'd replace old siding or update a faucet), we can still take precautions that allow our hearts to work well for as long as possible. If you take care of your house, it can last a long time.

Your race and ethnicity can also impact your risk. For example, African American and Native American individuals are more likely to develop heart disease. Certain racial and ethnic groups are more prone to some causes of heart disease such as high blood pressure, diabetes, and obesity—and these groups may have limited access to quality healthcare.[1]

Lastly, family history always plays a role in your risk. If you take two people who both have the same symptoms, experience the same issue, and receive the same treatment, there's always the chance that one will recover with no problems while the other may need further treatment and suffer more complications. The interesting thing about risk factors and genetic predisposition is that a patient can have all of the risk factors and not experience any heart issues. How many times have you gone to family gatherings and heard, "Look at Cousin Joe. With all the fatty foods he eats and the way he smokes, it won't surprise me if he keels over of a heart attack right here. Just look at how young his dad was when he died." But, despite all the dire predictions, Cousin Joe lives to the ripe old age of 92.

On the other hand, a patient can have no risk factors and still have a heart attack, like Aunt Cindy, the family health fanatic who had a mild heart attack during her daily 5-mile run. It all depends on genetic makeup, family history, and your body. You and your cardiologist must work together so you can be as healthy as possible in the situation in which you find yourself.

Modifiable Risk Factors

Whether or not you have non-modifiable risk factors, understanding those things you can control is a crucial component of the Artisan's Approach™. Knowing what makes you more susceptible to heart disease is the first step toward being an active participant in your health. Most of the literature geared toward the average consumer focuses on the risk factors for your heart's plumbing. The truth is, many of the same risky behaviors affect every area of the heart. While I'll talk about the risk factors that impact each part of your heart in the coming sections of this book, this chapter can serve as your slimmed-down cheat sheet.

Our hearts are no different than our houses: Some of us fill them with junk, while others take good care of them. Your diet plays a huge role in your heart health. If you're overeating or not eating enough healthy foods, you're at risk for obesity, diabetes, and, of course, heart disease. The biggest "no-nos" are sugary, greasy, and high-cholesterol foods, which all encourage plaque buildup in your arteries and put unnecessary strain on your heart.

Cholesterol—The Good and the Bad

Cholesterol is a waxy substance that circulates through your blood, and when you have too much of it, it can cause *plaque* to build up in your arteries. (Plaque is a substance that can accumulate on the inner walls of your arteries; when this happens, your arteries become clogged, which reduces blood flow.) For decades, high cholesterol has been painted as a villain when it comes to heart health, but it's not quite as simple as "all cholesterol is bad." Not all cholesterol is created alike. *Low-density lipoprotein (LDL)*, known as "bad cholesterol," sticks to the blood, clogging your arteries; but *high-density lipoprotein (HDL)* can benefit your heart health. Known as "good cholesterol," HDL helps remove bad cholesterol, fats, and plaque from your blood, and carries them to the liver to be cleared out of your system—it can reduce plaque buildup in your arteries! So, the issue isn't having high cholesterol in general, but having high LDL and not enough HDL.

> *I like to see total cholesterol below 200, the LDL below 100, and the HDL above 40 (for men) or 50 (for women).*

Your body gets cholesterol from two places: food and your liver. Dietary cholesterol, found in meat and other animal products, can raise the amount of cholesterol in your body, as can eating a diet high in saturated fat, which prompts the liver to produce more cholesterol. But, eating a heart-healthy diet low in saturated fat and high in fiber can lower your cholesterol, particularly the dangerous LDL, as well as help boost your HDL. Refraining from smoking and engaging in regular exercise can also raise your good cholesterol.

Diet

Countless books have been written on the topic of the foods we consume—and for good reason: Much of your health can be controlled through what you eat. Your diet can hurt you or help you. It's your choice. In the best scenario, your diet is a preventive measure. A heart-healthy diet focuses on a few key factors: It includes reasonable portions, is low in sodium, unhealthy fat, sugar, processed foods, and cholesterol, and is high in fruits and vegetables. In the worst-case scenario, if you overeat and consume too much sodium, unhealthy fat, sugar, processed food—and everything else that's not heart-healthy—you may eventually pay the price with heart disease.

Exercise

Even individuals with healthy diets are more likely to develop heart disease when they don't get enough exercise. Our bodies are made to move. Without exercise, your risk is similar to that of someone with high blood pressure (*hypertension*). So, even if you eat a perfect diet and have no other risk factors, without exercise, you might as well have high blood pressure.

> *Instead of taking a pill to lose weight, get active.*

Stress

Stress has a real physical effect on your body. We live in a world in which we're always rushed, trying to do more and more. This constant stress acts against your health, causing wear and tear on your heart. Emotional stress is the number one predictor of a heart attack. In fact, constantly elevated adrenaline wreaks havoc on most of the systems of your body. Pay attention to your stress and make managing it a priority. In Sanskrit, *pranayama* means "one breath"—in essence, "one life." If you don't take a breath, your entire body will cease to function. The heart can keep ticking, but if the breath is gone, you can't save that person.

Drugs, Coffee and Alcohol

The types of drugs you take and the frequency in which you use them also affect your chances of heart disease. Statistically, men are more likely to partake in risky behaviors such as excess alcohol and drug use, though drugs contribute to heart disease in both men and women. Stimulant drugs can be very dangerous to your electrical system, throwing off the heart's ability to pump. Stimulants range from very mild varieties like the caffeine in coffee to very dangerous substances like cocaine. Coffee in small doses will not significantly increase your risk of heart disease, and can benefit your health thanks to the antioxidants it contains; but, too much can be harmful.

Up to 400 mg of caffeine (the amount contained in about four cups of coffee) per day is generally considered safe for healthy adults.[2] However, it's important to note that some coffees and espresso-based drinks (such as many of those sold at Starbucks) contain much more caffeine than the average homebrew, and you can easily hit the upper limit with just one grande beverage. Also, if you have high blood pressure or are taking certain medications, you may not be able to tolerate as much caffeine.

It should go without saying that more frequent or harder drug use can mean damage to your health or even a death sentence. Even some prescription stimulants, like diet pills and decongestants, can be dangerous if you use them too much.

> *Think about what you're putting in your body and whether the short-term benefits outweigh the long-term damage!*

Alcohol is a curious substance. Limited use can help clean out your plumbing system (like Drano helps to clear the pipes in your house) because it raises your good cholesterol. So, drinking a fifth of whiskey should leave your arteries as clean as a whistle, right? You know I'm going to caution you otherwise, so no need to get your hopes up. Just as Drano can start to damage the porcelain of your sink or even the copper of your pipes if you use too much, excessive alcohol consumption can harm your heart. It will sweep through your pipes and clear them out, but you may also be doing irreparable damage to your heart's muscle or electrical system.

How much is too much? While it depends on your other risk factors, women should stick to one drink per day and men should limit themselves to two drinks. (A drink is considered 12 ounces of beer, 5 ounces of wine, or a 1.5-ounce shot of distilled spirits such as vodka, tequila or whiskey.)[3]

As with all aspects of your heart health, one recommendation doesn't fit all, however. For example, you may be one of those people whose heart's plumbing system might benefit from moderate amounts of both caffeine and alcohol, but whose heart's electrical system could be severely harmed by even the tiniest amount of either substance. This is why an individualized Artisan's Approach™ to caring for your heart is so important: You need doctors who take into consideration your unique situation and give you recommendations that are customized to reduce your particular risk.

Smoking

While I'm putting a damper on some readers' ideas of pleasurable pastimes, I should also address smoking. Unlike moderate alcohol use for most people, smoking—even a minimal amount—can do serious damage to your heart health. The harmful chemicals in cigarette smoke can encourage the buildup of plaque in your arteries; if you smoked for even a short time in your life, you may have accumulated dangerous plaque as a result. Some people argue that smoking calms their nerves, but what it really does is increase your blood pressure— bumping up your risk for heart disease even further—and feed your nicotine addiction.

Illnesses

Lastly, some illness and infections may suddenly trigger heart disease. These include, but aren't limited to, *Lyme carditis* (a complication of Lyme disease), *valve endocarditis* (an infection of the valves of the heart), *myocarditis* and *rheumatic fever* (a consequence of untreated strep infection that can cause heart valve damage). However, any severe illness will increase your risk for complications within your heart.

Risk factors are just that: factors that play a part in how likely you are to develop heart disease. There's no hard and fast rule that will help you avoid heart disease altogether or predict, without a doubt, that you will develop it. That said, when you take good care of yourself, your heart becomes healthier.

CHAPTER 4

The Cardiologist as General Contractor

"So, Doc, are you a plumber, an electrician, or a butcher?"

That was the question posed to me by a new patient, John, when I began practicing cardiology in Utah. Believe it or not, we cardiologists often refer to ourselves as plumbers and electricians (but certainly not butchers). Remember my Heart House analogy from the last chapter? When you want to build or maintain your home, you call in different specialists—for example, a plumber or an electrician—depending on your needs. It's the same in the world of cardiology: We have generalists, and we have specialists who focus on particular heart conditions.

General cardiologists are the primary care providers of cardiology. Your primary care doctor may refer you to a cardiologist. My job is akin to that of a general contractor. It's my responsibility to know everything happening inside your heart. Much like a general contractor for your home, I understand the plumbing and electrical systems, as well as the construction design and materials so that I can monitor and detect any current or potential problems. To do this, I conduct a physical examination, run some tests, and perhaps use advanced imaging technology. Once I determine the issue (or issues), I treat you or, if necessary, refer you to an appropriate subcontractor for treatment; it's a team approach.

I enjoy being a generalist because I get to care for my patients for the rest of their lives, helping them first to achieve heart health and then maintain it. I also get the opportunity to work with an amazing team of expert specialists who consistently provide support, guidance, and insight for our patients. I rely heavily on their authority and expertise to create the best treatment plans possible.

Back to John: I replied, "I'm a clown who keeps you happy and does part-time photography." Understandably, patients sitting on the other side of my desk are often gloomy and fearful of hearing the worst. I use my skills as an artisan, attempting to lighten the mood as I deliver what is often somber information.

I call myself a part-time photographer because much of my job involves diagnosing patients through cardiac imaging: using equipment that takes pictures of the heart. Taking pictures of the heart is an integral part of how I diagnose and care for patients as a board-certified multimodality advanced imaging specialist.

Let's take a look at some of the specialists a cardiac patient might need. Each doctor on your team has a vital role in diagnosing, treating, and managing the care of your heart.

- The "plumber" (*interventional cardiologist*) is a specialist who diagnoses and treats problems in the blood vessels and cardiovascular system of your heart.
- The "electrician" (*cardiac electrophysiologist*) works specifically with the rhythm of your heart, diagnosing and treating heart rhythm abnormalities.
- The "carpenter" (*cardiothoracic or cardiovascular surgeon*) is in charge of the surgical treatment of your heart, including common procedures such as bypasses and valve replacements. As a bonus, the cardiovascular surgeon is often trained to perform surgical procedures on the lungs, esophagus, and other organs in the chest.
- The "photographer" (*cardiac imaging specialist*) performs and interprets cardiac imaging studies like echocardiograms, nuclear stress tests, cardiac PET (Positron Emission Tomography) scans, cardiac MRI, and CT coronary angiography.

Hopefully, you've never had reason to think about—much less meet with—all the different kinds of cardiac specialists that exist. But isn't it comforting to know that there's a virtual smorgasbord of highly trained experts out there who are qualified to work with your exact problem if you need them? (Take a look at the chart at the end of this chapter for an overview of five types of cardiology specialists.) Getting back to my favorite comparison, think of these physicians like the professionals you'd call when purchasing or renovating your house. When you're buying a house, you bring in an inspector. Like a general contractor, he's knowledgeable in all aspects of construction (in fact, many inspectors have also worked as general contractors), and his job is to tell you everything that may be wrong with the house. If, instead of a general inspector, you brought in a plumber, he might only see the problems with the plumbing and miss the faulty electrical wires. Or, if you brought in a mason, he might only see the problems with the brick and miss the leaking pipes. This exemplifies why having a general inspector and contractor who can be both objective and thorough is invaluable. That's the job of a general cardiologist.

Similarly, if you were renovating your house, you wouldn't call a plumber to fix an electrical issue, nor would you call an electrician to replace the doors. Each specialist focuses on the single area in which they're an expert. As a general contractor, I'm only as good as the subcontractors I work with. Each member of the team has a unique role in the management of your heart health. Without a solid team, my patients would receive a lower quality of care. (That said, there are several heart issues that general cardiologists treat without the need to refer the patient to a specialist, including high blood pressure, the most common cardiovascular condition.)

Cardiology specialists and subspecialists all see your heart condition through the lens of their training and specializations, which is why becoming an involved and informed patient is so important. A doctor who's spent decades fixing issues in the plumbing of the heart will want to jump in and fix plumbing issues first, whereas I may look at the big picture and suggest holding off on that to address more pressing health matters. I know I'm getting redundant here, but this particular point is worth stressing many times over: A better-educated patient will be better able to understand the various aspects of their care and participate in deciding the "best" course of action.

It takes an army of nurses, primary cardiologists, specialists, and equipment to successfully understand, diagnose, treat, and manage cardiac conditions. Each person on the team has measureless value within your support system. All are highly educated and trained to play a specific role in caring for your heart. Although each one analyzes your heart from a different perspective, it is this diversity that provides well-rounded and needed care.

Cardiology Professionals

Specialty	Basic Job Description	Primary Roles
General Cardiologist ("The General Contractor")	The chief cardiac caregiver who sees the patient on an ongoing basis	• Diagnoses and treats common conditions such as hypertension (high blood pressure) and high cholesterol • Refers the patient to subspecialists as needed for non-routine care • Coordinates care among multiple cardiac subspecialists
Interventional Cardiologist ("The Plumber")	Treats/resolves issues with the heart and blood vessels using catheter-based procedures[1]	• Performs procedures to open narrowed/blocked blood vessels
Cardiac Electrophysiologist ("The Electrician")	Diagnoses and treats heart rhythm abnormalities	Implants pacemakers, inserts defibrillators, and performs other procedures to correct heart rhythm problems
Cardiothoracic Surgeon ("The Carpenter")	Provides surgical treatment for heart problems	Performs coronary artery bypass grafts (CABGs), valve repair/replacement, and heart transplants
Cardiac Imaging Specialist ("The Photographer")	Performs and interprets cardiac imaging tests	Performs cardiac imaging studies such echocardiogram, nuclear stress tests, cardiac PET (Positron Emission Tomography) scans, cardiac MRI, and CT coronary angiography.

---

[1] Cather-based procedures involve threading a thin, flexible tube through the blood vessels.

CHAPTER 5

Diagnosing Heart Problems

When diagnosing a heart problem, the first thing I do is take the patient's medical history. This begins before I walk into the patient's room as my nurse or medical assistant gathers some basic information on the patient's medical background, medications they're taking, and the reason for the visit. The nurse or assistant also takes the patient's vital signs, including their blood pressure and pulse, measures height and weight, and prints copies of any recent bloodwork.

All of this information helps me begin to take an Artisan's Approach™ to caring for the patient, even before I begin my exam. Once I enter the exam room, I begin by asking questions including:

- What are your symptoms?
- Do you have a family history of heart problems?
- Have you ever been diagnosed with high blood pressure?
- Have you been sick lately?
- Have you received any medical treatments?
- Have you taken any drugs?

After completing the history, I do a thorough physical examination and listen to the patient's heart with my *stethoscope.* Everyone who's ever visited a doctor has seen a stethoscope draped around the doctor's neck.

The stethoscope has been around for more than 200 years! Before its invention, physicians positioned their ear directly on a patient's chest. In 1816, Dr. René Laennec of Paris, France was uncomfortable placing his ear on the chest of an overweight woman. Instead, he rolled up a sheet of paper into a tube, put one end of the tube on her chest, and discovered the sounds were magnified. The stethoscope was invented![1]

My stethoscope provides me with some useful information: It allows me to hear signs of trouble including "whooshing" noises, a heartbeat that's irregular or fast, and even crackling sounds.

In most cases, I order the same diagnostic tests: those that will help provide answers about heart issues and symptoms. These tests include an EKG, bloodwork, and chest X-rays. Then, depending on the patient's circumstances, I commonly order an echocardiogram and a stress test. Except for the bloodwork, these tests are *noninvasive,* meaning no instruments are inserted into your body. The results of these tests help me to determine next steps and if more advanced tests are needed. They may also reveal that a patient's symptoms are stemming from something other than heart issues. Let's take a closer look at some of these tests.

Electrocardiogram

An *electrocardiogram (EKG)*[2] measures the electrical impulses of your heart. While this test won't tell your doctor the exact cause of your problems, an EKG is often the first test we order because it's fairly straightforward. A physician, nurse, or technician attaches sticky patches embedded with electrodes to your chest. These electrodes read the electrical signals that fire as your heart pumps, and then transmit that information to a monitor, which charts your heart's activity on graph paper. An EKG is painless, takes only five minutes, and doesn't require any special preparation. To most people, an electrocardiogram tracing looks like a bunch of random peaks, hills, and valleys. In reality, these peaks, hills, and valleys represent the electrical activity of your heart and follow very specific patterns. Normal EKG results suggest that nothing is critically wrong with the heart muscle. In patients with heart issues, we see variations from a normal EKG reading.

Bloodwork

Your blood provides many clues to your heart health, including your risk for having a heart attack. The standard tests for heart issues include:

- Total cholesterol.
- *Low-density lipoprotein* (LDL) cholesterol (the "bad" cholesterol).
- *High-density lipoprotein* (HDL) cholesterol (the "good" cholesterol).

---

[2] The British abbreviation for electrocardiogram is ECG, while the American abbreviation is EKG.

- *Triglycerides*, a type of fat in the blood.
- *High-sensitivity C-reactive protein* (*hsCRP*), a sign of inflammation in the body. This test alone doesn't necessarily point to heart disease, but combined with other test results, it helps to provide a picture of your overall heart health.

There are additional blood tests that can help diagnose a heart problem, but these are the standard ones.

Chest X-Rays

A *chest X-ray* creates pictures of the structures inside your chest using electromagnetic waves. These X-rays show the size and shape of your heart and the outline of your heart's large arteries and veins, and can even detect the presence of calcium in your heart.

Exercise Stress Test

The *exercise stress test*, also called a *treadmill stress test*, or just a *stress test*, enables a doctor to evaluate your heart's performance during physical activity. First, the doctor or technician measures your blood pressure and heart rate (pulse) and takes an EKG reading of your heart at rest. Then, all these things are monitored while you walk on a treadmill or pedal a stationary bicycle with increasing intensity, to see how your heart keeps up with the growing demand of physical activity, and how it recovers after you slow down or stop moving. Many heart issues that aren't apparent during rest, like an irregular heartbeat, are easy to see during a stress test. If you're not able to walk or pedal for whatever reason, medications may be used to "stress" your heart and make it respond as it would to real activity. This is called a *pharmacological stress test* or *adenosine* or *dobutamine stress test*.

Echocardiogram

Often the most telling tests doctors conduct on patients with potential heart problems is the *echocardiogram*, sometimes shortened to "echo" or "cardiac echo." An echocardiogram is a type of ultrasound test that sends harmless sound waves into your chest, which then reflect back so the machine can create a picture. The same technology is used to "see" babies in the womb. The waves create a moving picture of your heart walls and how they function in real time.

Numerous tests can help doctors determine what's going on in your heart and the best strategies for enabling you to achieve heart health. But tests alone don't result in a good treatment plan. These tests are tools, and it takes an Artisan's Approach™ to interpret them in light of your unique situation.

PART 3

The Circulation: Your Heart's Plumbing System

CHAPTER 6

How the Circulation Works

Running through the interior and exterior walls of your house, unseen behind the drywall, is an intricate system of pipes carrying water to all of the sinks, toilets, and showers in your house, as well as the dishwasher and washing machine. There's another set of pipes that leads from all these items out of the house.

A similar system runs throughout your heart. Within its walls is your heart's plumbing: These arteries (*coronary arteries*) and veins (*cardiac veins*) supply oxygenated blood to the heart, and return deoxygenated blood to the lungs to pick up more oxygen. And, just like a plumbing problem in your home can wreak havoc on other parts of the house (flooding and leaks in your ceiling, for example), an issue with the plumbing of your heart can impact other aspects of your cardiac health.

You could say the heart has two circulatory systems: one that provides blood flow to the heart itself (coronary artery system), and another that pumps blood out to the entire body (the aorta and its branches). Our focus in this section of the book is the coronary artery system, the plumbing of the heart itself.

If you were to open up the walls of your house, you'd find one simple pipe, appropriately named the water main, which supplies your entire house with clean, fresh water. From this larger pipe, smaller pipes branch out, taking water to various destinations throughout the home. Like your house's water main, the heart has one main artery that serves a similar function: the aorta. Instead of carrying water, however, the aorta handles the blood that courses throughout your body. Other pipes, or arteries, split off from the aorta and serve specific functions. The coronary artery system, which includes the left and right coronary arteries, is the first side branch off the aorta. We'll take a look at the aorta in more detail in Part 8.

If you're unfamiliar with plumbing, the sight of all those pipes behind your house's walls, weaving in and out, circling corners, and connecting with other pipes may appear as confusing as traveling through an endless maze. A full discussion of the coronary arteries can be equally overwhelming, so I'll spare you most of it! But, here's a key concept about your heart's plumbing that you should understand:

The *right and left coronary arteries* branch off the aorta, transporting blood to the heart itself.

- The right coronary artery (RCA) supplies blood to the right side of the heart (via the right ventricle) and bottom of the heart.

- The left coronary artery (also called the left main coronary artery) supplies blood to the rest of the heart via its two major branches: the *left anterior descending (LAD) artery* and the *left circumflex artery (LCX)*.

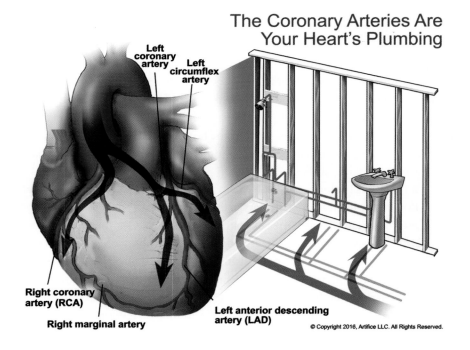

The Coronary Arteries Are Your Heart's Plumbing

Left coronary artery

Left circumflex artery

Right coronary artery (RCA)

Right marginal artery

Left anterior descending artery (LAD)

© Copyright 2016, Artifice LLC. All Rights Reserved.

Again, there's a lot more to the heart's plumbing, but it's complicated. Remembering the following points will help you understand ensuing discussions:

1. The coronary arteries supply blood to the heart itself. Problems in these arteries are serious: If the flow of oxygen and nutrients to the heart itself is slowed down or blocked, it can lead to a heart attack or death. Disease of the coronary arteries is aptly named *coronary artery disease (CAD)*.

2. Since the LAD artery is responsible for transporting blood to a large portion of the left ventricle, blockages in the LAD can be particularly dangerous. You may have heard of the "widow maker." Well, this is it. When this main artery is completely blocked or has a significant blockage at the beginning (where it connects to the aorta), the entire artery after it goes down—causing a massive heart attack that will likely lead to sudden death, thus the term "widow maker."

The coronary artery system is the plumbing of the heart itself. It includes the left and right coronary arteries, and is the first side branch off the aorta, which supplies the entire body with blood.

CHAPTER 7

Circulation Problems and Symptoms

Like every other muscle in your body, your heart needs a steady supply of oxygen-rich blood to function. When the pipes that send blood to your heart become narrowed or blocked altogether, it can't do its job and the results can be disastrous.

Coronary Artery Disease

Every Taco Tuesday for years, you've stood at your kitchen sink and strained the extra fat from your cooked ground beef right down the drain. You know that isn't the way you're supposed to deal with excess grease, but you haven't given it a second thought—until today. For the past few weeks, you've noticed that water hasn't been draining as quickly as normal, but you've chalked it up to a bean or some other item of food being stuck in the drain, and have been sure it would wash down eventually. But today, water is backing up in your sink, and the drain seems to be partially blocked. While you decide to call the plumber before the drain clogs completely, someone else might wait until the sink is completely stopped up. In either case, the plumber comes and finds years of hardened, greasy buildup that's preventing water from flowing freely. Depending on the damage, either he unclogs the drainage pipes with a plumbing snake or replaces them with new pipes, then charges a hefty fee for his services. All that ground beef fat can add up.

When you hear people talking about stenosis, roto rooter, angina, chest pain, balloon stent, and bypasses, they're talking about the heart's plumbing problems.

A clogged pipe in your Heart House works in a similar fashion: When your coronary arteries are healthy, your blood flows freely. But, in diseased coronary arteries, a substance called *plaque* builds up inside your artery walls. When most people hear the word plaque, they think of the gross stuff their dental hygienist scrapes off their teeth. Of course, plaque buildup in the arteries is quite different than the plaque on your teeth, but both are pretty disgusting. Arterial plaque is made of fat, cholesterol, and other substances found in the blood, and is very dangerous. In fact, most problems with your heart's plumbing stem from this buildup of plaque, which we call *atherosclerosis*. If you have atherosclerosis, this buildup of plaque, you have *coronary artery disease.* Over time, this plaque buildup becomes calcified, meaning it accumulates calcium.

Be aware that atherosclerosis isn't the same as *arteriosclerosis*, the stiffening or hardening of the artery walls from aging. Atherosclerosis is a specific type of arteriosclerosis. Rest assured, these two terms confuse even the brightest medical students—but both conditions can result in dangers to your health.

Artery with and without Plaque

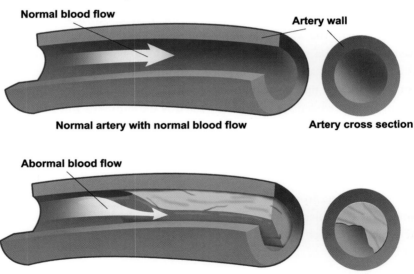

Normal blood flow

Artery wall

Normal artery with normal blood flow

Artery cross section

Abormal blood flow

Artery with plaque buildup

Narrowed artery

Just like the clog in your kitchen sink can impair the movement of water through the pipes, the buildup in your heart's plumbing can result in reduced blood flow. Over time, the plaque increases, hardens, and bulges inward, causing your arteries to narrow. In the medical world, we use the term *"stenosis"* to refer to an abnormal narrowing of any channel in the body. The inside space of your arteries is called the lumen, so the narrowing of your arteries is called *luminal stenosis*—but I'll keep it simple and just say "stenosis. "

Years of Taco Tuesdays, among other indulgences, can exact a very painful toll.

Two Types of Plaque: Stable and Unstable

At first, you hear a faint clank or two. You wonder what's causing it, but not enough to investigate. After all, the house isn't new, and peculiar creaks, groans, and banging sounds are to be expected. But it becomes louder and more prominent, particularly when you turn on the water, and the noises are becoming harder and harder to ignore. Time to call in a plumber and make sure there's nothing serious going on. You don't want any pipes to rupture or become blocked again. You call in the same professional who removed the clog in your drain; he examines the pipes and explains you have a couple of types of buildup inside.

You've already learned that your arteries can develop buildup called plaque. Plaque contains two parts: a core and a soft, fibrous cap. Both the plaque and the fibrous cap may be thick or thin. And, there are two types of plaque. One is prone to rupture, and the other is not:

1. *Stable plaque,* made of a calcium-rich core with a strong, thick fibrous cap, is unlikely to rupture. (Calcium is a hard substance, which makes the plaque more stable.)
2. *Unstable plaque (*also known as *vulnerable plaque),* is made of a fat-rich core with a thin cap. Unstable plaque is more likely to rupture because of its soft core and thin cap.

Stable plaque can sit silently in your arteries for many years before it presents any symptoms. Although the presence of stable plaque is a serious issue, it often can be detected and treated over a period of time. However, when it comes to unpredictable danger, unstable (vulnerable) plaque is the super villain. This hard-to-detect plaque buildup doesn't obstruct the blood flow through your arteries, yet it causes the majority of all heart attacks.[1] Unstable plaque hidden in the walls of the heart can rupture suddenly, resulting in an acute (sudden) heart attack.

Stable Versus Unstable Plaque

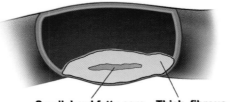

Small, hard fatty core   Thick, fibrous cap

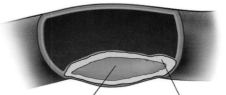

Large, soft fatty core   This, fibrous cap

Two Types of Coronary Artery Disease: Obstructive and Non-Obstructive

Stable plaque builds slowly inside your artery walls and progresses over the years to cause stenosis, a narrowing of the artery. If the plaque buildup grows large enough inside your artery walls, at a certain point (usually when the artery is about 70% blocked), it will reduce the blood flow to your heart. Since this condition obstructs the blood flow to your heart, it's known as *obstructive coronary artery disease*. If you have stable plaque that's not impeding blood flow to your heart (typically less than a 70% narrowing of the artery), we call it *non-obstructive coronary artery disease,* or just atherosclerosis.

I tell my patients that reduced blood flow to the heart causes the heart muscle to "cry out in pain," and we call this pain *angina,* a term that simply means discomfort or pain in the chest. *Stable angina* (also called *classic angina),* is predictable in that the chest pain occurs only with a certain amount of activity or stress.

Narrowed arteries may function sufficiently at rest, but can't keep up with the increased amount of oxygenated blood that's delivered to the heart during physical exertion, like climbing stairs. If you can predict that certain activities will trigger chest pain, you're probably experiencing stable angina, which will pass after you rest or take medication.

Angina isn't a disease; rather, it's a sign of an underlying issue—such as atherosclerosis. In addition to chest pain, symptoms of stable angina may include shortness of breath, fatigue, jaw pain, and left arm pain. Sometimes angina feels exactly like indigestion.

Before you jump to the conclusion that the discomfort you feel is related to stable angina, you should know that other conditions can also cause chest pain. These include indigestion, heartburn or acid reflux, gallstones, muscle sprains, and other heart-related issues. So, while chest pain is often a sign of coronary artery disease, that's not always the case. Although stable angina isn't necessarily an emergency condition, it does indicate underlying heart disease that makes a heart attack more likely for you than for someone without angina. It should serve as a powerful warning to improve your lifestyle: quit smoking, lose weight, get active, and stop the Taco Tuesdays, even if Mexican is your favorite cuisine. Your heart is telling you it's starving for better blood flow. It's obviously better to respond to the angina in the hopes of preventing a heart attack than to give in to your cravings.

> ***Don't play a guessing game when it comes to your life.***
> ***If you have chest pain, get to your doctor and have it checked out.***

Taking note of and discussing your symptoms with your doctor can help you come up with a plan to reduce these incidents, treat them when they occur, and distinguish these pains from the kind of chest pains that should prompt you to call 911 immediately.

Heart Attacks

It Was So Unexpected!

Scott spent most of his days working in the warm sun, keeping his grapevines healthy and his farm productive. Ten years prior, he'd left his desk job and purchased a beautiful 100-acre winery with his wife. On a day that was indistinguishable from any other, Scott was tending to his grapes when he felt a sudden pain shoot through his chest. He clutched his heart and collapsed.

At age 45, Scott had had a heart attack. It took Scott totally by surprise, and his family echoed those sentiments:

"He's always been so healthy!" said Scott's brother.

"It was so unexpected," sobbed Scott's wife.

Indeed, Scott had always gone for yearly physical exams, kept his weight in a healthy range, and had never been found to have high blood pressure. So why was he now in the emergency room?

Alas, once doctors thoroughly examined Scott and performed some tests, the answer was clear: A super villain had been lurking dormant in his arteries for years, just waiting for the perfect chance to strike. In one completely unexpected twist of fate, his vulnerable plaque had ruptured, causing Scott to fall to the ground as those around him looked on in disbelief—and proving that no one is entirely immune from the possibility of a heart attack.

So, what exactly is a *heart attack*? Simply put, it's damage to an area of your heart that's deprived of oxygen, usually because of a blocked artery. *Myocardial infarction* (literally, "death of the heart muscle"), is the medical term for a heart attack. However, among ourselves, we doctors use a newer term, *ACS* or *acute coronary syndrome*, an umbrella term for a range of conditions in which blood flow to the heart is suddenly blocked or reduced.

Unlike stable angina, which is predictable and happens only with activity, the symptoms of a heart attack usually come on *suddenly* while a person is *at rest* and include:

- Chest pain or discomfort
- Pain or discomfort in the jaw, neck, back, stomach, or arms
- Indigestion
- Vomiting
- Shortness of breath
- Sweating
- Feeling dizzy or lightheaded

As an artisan, one of my objectives is to explain the heart and how it functions in language that anyone can comprehend. Here's my Artisan's Approach™ to helping you understand what happens during a heart attack:

	What Happens	**Medical Term**
1.	An artery gets blocked	Luminal stenosis
2.	The heart doesn't get enough oxygen	Myocardial ischemia
3.	The person experiences pain as the heart muscle cries out	Angina
4.	The heart cells begin to die	Myocardial infarction or heart attack

Unstable Angina, NSTEMI, and STEMI

There are three types of heart attacks, each resulting from clogged arteries: *unstable angina* (less serious), *NSTEMI* (somewhat serious), and *STEMI* (most serious). The differences between the three types of heart attack stem from the amount of damage to your heart, and the severity of blockage in your arteries. As the patient, you just know you've had a heart attack. But, doctors treat you differently depending on which type of heart attack you've had. I know all of this doctor lingo can be a bit much. As an artisan, I strive to keep it simple for my patients, so I just say "heart attack," and for the most part, that's the term I'll use in this book. However, I'd like my readers to become familiar with terms (such as ACS, unstable angina, NSTEMI, and STEMI) that may appear in their medical records, and also to know what type of heart attack they've been treated for. Perhaps my explanation will help you next time you view your medical records, or receive a hospital bill or Medicare statement, and you won't feel like you're drowning in medical jargon.

As you recall, stable angina is predictable chest pain due to a significant plaque buildup in your heart's artery, which causes stenosis or obstruction, and therefore a lack of blood flow. We call this obstruction *myocardial ischemia*. The word *ischemia* refers to the restriction of blood supply to any organ or tissue in the body, including the heart. Myocardial ischemia simply refers to a lack of oxygen to the heart due to narrowed arteries.

No one is immune from a heart attack. Jim Fixx, the American author of *The Complete Book of Running,* was at the forefront of a health and fitness movement that spread throughout the United States in the 1970s, and continued to flourish in the decades since his rise to fame. An avid jogger, he collapsed and died of a heart attack while on a routine run at the age of 52. An autopsy revealed that atherosclerosis had blocked three of his coronary arteries.

On the other hand, heart attacks are caused by a sudden obstruction of blood flow from ruptured unstable (vulnerable) plaque, and are unpredictable: They usually come on suddenly—while you're sleeping or resting, or with just a little exertion. Contrary to what many people believe, heart attacks are not caused by arteries that have been narrowed by plaque!

Picture the beautiful islands of Hawaii, full of lush green plants, exotic wildlife, and of course, beautiful beaches. Beneath this picturesque landscape lies a maze of underground lava channels. The lava isn't dangerous for the people or animals living on the islands because they're protected by layers of rock and earth. But when the density and pressure build within the lava, it will explode out of the volcano. What was once dormant and harmless now causes extensive damage as it burns and hardens. Unstable plaque can act similarly: It may remain silent for a long time, offering no clues that it's there—no pain, no symptoms at all—and it doesn't even show up on a stress test. We live our lives in blissful couch potato indulgence—hacking our way through a pack-a-day or more habit, devouring giant burgers with all the fixings, never turning down that last piece of cake—unaware of the developing risk until one day ... kaboom! The plaque ruptures, filling our arteries.

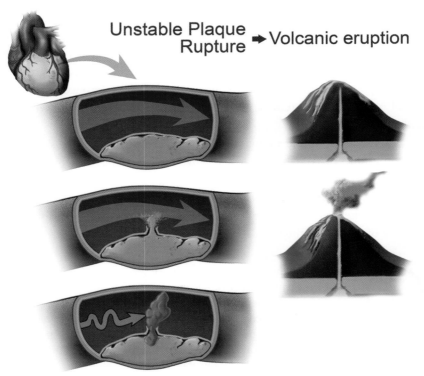

Unstable Plaque Rupture ➡ Volcanic eruption

When unstable plaque volcanically erupts, your body responds just like it does when you get a cut and your body forms a scab: It sends platelets to form a blood clot. The medical term for blood clot is *thrombus*, and the formation of a blood clot that blocks an artery is called *thrombosis*. The two main components of blood clots are *fibrin*, a strong protein, and *platelets*, a type of blood cell. Fibrin and platelets work together to stop a blood clot from falling apart. Depending on where it forms, this clot can quickly block blood flow to your heart. This is how sudden and severe heart attacks occur.

About 70% of heart attack patients have either unstable angina or an NSTEMI.[2] These conditions are sometimes lumped together because they're treated similarly.

When a patient reports to the emergency room with chest pain, it can be difficult to tell which one they're experiencing from their symptoms alone. We determine if a heart attack is caused by unstable angina or an NSTEMI using a blood test that checks for certain markers of heart damage, called *cardiac biomarkers*. (More on biomarkers in a few pages.) If the biomarkers are elevated, indicating damage to the heart cells, the diagnosis is an NSTEMI; if the biomarkers aren't elevated, it's unstable angina.

Problems in your heart's plumbing system are caused by a buildup of plaque. This plaque can be stable or unstable. Stable plaque can grow large enough to obstruct the blood flow to the heart muscle, causing stable angina.

Heart attacks are caused by the volcanic eruption of unstable plaque. The three types of heart attacks are unstable angina, NSTEMI, and STEMI.

CHAPTER 8

Causes of Circulation Problems

In Chapter 3, we talked in general about some of the causes of heart disease, but let's look specifically at the causes of your heart's plumbing problems. In a word, the main problem is plaque. Some individuals are more prone to developing plaque buildup than others. While some risk factors for plaque are out of doctors' and patients' control, others are impacted by lifestyle.

The older you are, the more likely you are to acquire plaque buildup over your lifetime, and the more likely it is that this plaque will narrow your arteries and restrict blood flow. If you think about the plumbing in your house, a similar mechanism is at play: Over time, wear and tear take place and after a while (particularly if you haven't done some regular maintenance), some of the plumbing may stop functioning optimally and need repair.

However, plaque is preventable, so please do something about it! Stop smoking, eat your fruits and veggies, consume alcohol in moderation, get moving, and take control of your weight, your cholesterol, and your blood pressure!

Men and women have somewhat different risks for plumbing problems. Men are more likely to have issues at a younger age than women, but women can catch up quickly once they pass through menopause, particularly if they didn't take good care of themselves when they were younger.

High cholesterol also puts you at risk, but it's a byproduct of poor lifestyle choices such as smoking, being overweight or obese, high blood pressure, physical inactivity, and stress.

However, some people have lived extremely healthy lifestyles and maintained healthy diets, yet they still run into plumbing problems. They have what I refer to as bad luck. They might have been born with some genetic predisposition for heart disease that can cause problems, even if they maintain heart-healthy lifestyles. Sometimes these issues go undetected until they experience chest pain or have a heart attack. I certainly don't advocate that these individuals throw in the towel and binge on donuts—just the opposite. If you know your family has a bleak cardiac history, you should do everything you can to stave off trouble.

CHAPTER 9

Diagnosing Circulation Problems

As we discussed in Chapter 5, the standard procedure for diagnosing any heart problem includes:

- Taking a complete medical history.
- Doing a thorough physical exam.
- Ordering the standard tests.

Of course, there's a difference between a patient coming to my office complaining of occasional chest pain and someone arriving at the ER with severe chest pain.

Non-obstructive CAD

Remember: If you have stable plaque that's not impeding blood flow to your heart, we call it non-obstructive coronary artery disease, or just atherosclerosis. Until recently, we had no tools or tests to detect atherosclerosis or plaque before this condition caused significant stenosis and resulted in a reduced blood flow to the heart (myocardial ischemia).

Cardiac CT Scan

The *cardiac CT scan* is relatively new and has been a real game changer. Until the advent of this technology, cardiologists had no means of determining if "at risk" patients had non-obstructive CAD. The cardiac CT scan uses an X-ray machine to take detailed pictures of the heart. This painless procedure can quickly help detect numerous abnormalities in the heart. When it comes to diagnosing your heart's plumbing problems, the cardiac CT scan helps cardiologists detect and evaluate two things: calcium buildup in the walls of your arteries, and plaque—both stable and unstable. The detection of stable plaque allows cardiologists to intervene before there are any symptoms. And, since the cardiac CT scan helps us differentiate between stable and unstable plaque, we can more aggressively attack unstable plaque—and, hopefully, prevent volcanic eruptions in patients' coronary arteries that result in heart attacks.

Coronary Calcium Score

Your arteries should be free of calcium. Any calcium buildup in your heart's plumbing may be a sign of coronary artery disease that could eventually lead to a heart attack. A type of cardiac CT scan can detect calcium buildup, and we give the overall calcium presence a score—aptly called the *coronary calcium score*. The higher the calcium, the higher the risk of heart attack.

Cardiologists don't have a crystal ball to predict heart problems, but the cardiac CT scan provides information that can equip doctors and patients with knowledge and the ability to make changes that may improve a patient's future. For example, once a patient's calcium score is determined, I use my Artisan's Approach™ to tailor your treatment accordingly. A calcium score can help you and your doctor develop a preventive plan that could keep you safe from deadly CAD.

 Cardiologist Dr. Arthur Agatston, the developer of the South Beach Diet, invented the coronary calcium score.

Coronary CT Angiogram (CCTA)

The *coronary CT angiogram (CCTA)* assesses the coronary arteries and detects blockages. This test uses high-powered X-rays to produce images of your heart and its blood vessels, and is performed using the same scanner as the calcium score. The CT Angiogram uses an iodinated contrast (meaning an iodine-containing contrast dye is injected into an IV in the patient's arm) to improve the quality of the images. The entire test lasts 10 to 30 minutes.

Obstructive CAD

As we've discussed, obstructive CAD isn't necessarily an emergency condition, but it does indicate underlying heart disease that makes a heart attack more likely for you than for someone without angina. If activity brings on chest pain, your doctor will order tests to determine the extent of your heart disease and the steps that should be taken to prevent a heart attack. The test of choice for obstructive CAD is the *imaging stress test*. Similar to the exercise stress test, the imaging stress test provides images showing the blood flow to the heart at rest and during exercise. Types of imaging used in this test include the echocardiogram, PET scan, and Cardiac MRI. The stress test is named based on the sort of imaging that's used—for example, the echo stress test.

If patients can't use the treadmill (for various reasons including obesity or a neurological disorder such as Parkinson's), we give them a *pharmacological stress test:* The patient is given drugs that have the same effect on their heart as exercise.

Unstable or Vulnerable Plaque

Patients who have vulnerable plaque often appear healthy. Unfortunately, the standard tests such as EKGs, blood tests, echocardiograms, and even stress tests will not diagnose vulnerable plaques hidden in your heart's arteries. Patients might even pass their stress test with flying colors because the real danger lies under their artery walls. To detect vulnerable plaque, we use the cardiac CT scan, which detects the silent threat of vulnerable plaque with a high level of accuracy so it can be treated effectively.

Research has shown that aggressive treatment with a *statin* (medication that helps reduce bad cholesterol) can help prevent the plaque from rupturing. On the other hand, if patients visit their cardiologist regularly and don't show a risk for vulnerable plaque, we're able to monitor them without medicine. We don't want to put everyone on medicine when only some need it, and the CT scan helps us determine which patients are at high risk. This test allows us to predict future issues and aim preventive care toward the right people. And in this case, the right people are those who have unstable plaque. I sit down with each of these patients and make sure they understand what we're dealing with. I find that explaining the results using my volcanic eruption analogy, another example of my Artisan's Approach™, helps me create awareness of the risk factor. It's a simple approach that helps patients start taking their diet and exercise routines more seriously. If they have diabetes or hypertension, my patients seem to manage their problems more responsibly once they envision a volcanic eruption and see the plaque that's waiting to emerge. Of course, these images also inspire my patients to faithfully follow the aggressive treatment of aspirin and statins I prescribe to prevent heart attacks.

Judging from my patients' reactions, images speak much louder than words. It's the quickest way I know to grab a patient's attention—especially when paired with the volcanic eruption analogy. If you undergo an imaging test, ask for the images or have your doctor show them to you and explain what you're seeing. If images don't motivate you to buckle down and take your heart health seriously, I doubt anything will.

Heart Attacks

The First Order of Business: Diagnosis

Sam was having some chest pain, so his wife drove him to the hospital where I work. He walked into the ER and said he thought he was having a heart attack. After asking him a few brief questions, the ER doctor ordered an EKG and then asked me to go to the ER and check in on Sam. Since the EKG showed that Sam had an NSTEMI, we started him on blood thinners, and I told him he'd be transferred to our tertiary care hospital (specialized care hospital) the next morning for an angiogram—as long as he didn't experience any more symptoms and his heart rate and blood pressure remained stable. There was panic in his voice as he replied, "My brother-in-law was taken care of right away at another hospital. Why can't I go right in?"

The way doctors react to a heart attack depends largely on which type you're having. I had to explain to Sam the difference between a STEMI and an NSTEMI heart attack.

"You've had an NSTEMI, and I know that's frightening to you," I said, "but the type of heart attack you've had is less serious than another kind, the STEMI. While an NSTEMI is serious, and can result in some damage to the heart, a STEMI is much more critical because damage can occur very quickly. The EKG lets me know which kind of heart attack you've had, which artery is causing the issue, and whether your artery is completely blocked. Believe me, the fact that you're spending the night right here instead of being rushed elsewhere is a good sign."

When we suspect someone is having a heart attack, one of the very first things we do is order an electrocardiogram (EKG). In a healthy heart that beats normally, the tiny electrical charges (*depolarization*) that prompt the heart muscle to beat following an orderly pattern. Cardiologists look for various kinds of abnormalities in the rhythm when assessing a patient. When we suspect a heart attack, the first place we look on the EKG is an area called the ST segment. A STEMI heart attack results from a complete and prolonged blockage of an artery in the heart, and this blocked artery shows up as an abnormal, elevated ST line on the EKG. If a patient's EKG shows ST elevation, their blocked artery needs to be opened right away because they're at a significant risk of suffering cardiac arrest (when the heart stops beating altogether) and death. It's often thought that a heart attack and cardiac arrest are the same thing; they aren't. However, a heart attack can cause cardiac arrest and sudden death.

On the other hand, an EKG that doesn't show ST-segment elevation indicates that the patient has had an NSTEMI or unstable angina. This means blood flow is compromised, but not completely blocked. It's still a serious medical emergency, but it's not as bad as a STEMI. As I mentioned earlier, NSTEMIs and unstable angina together account for 70% of heart attacks. STEMI heart attacks account for about 30% of all heart attacks.[1]

If you call 911 and tell the emergency responder you have the symptoms of a heart attack, you'll be asked a series of questions and most likely will also be instructed to chew a baby aspirin (non-coated, 162 to 325 mg) right away. If you have nitroglycerin, the trained person on the other end of the line will advise you to take a dose immediately, in addition to the aspirin. Meanwhile, they'll order an ambulance. When you arrive at the ER complaining of chest pain and the staff suspects you may be having a heart attack, a protocol will be implemented immediately to ensure that, if you do have a blocked artery, it's diagnosed and fixed as soon as possible.

Sometimes, patients having STEMI heart attacks don't seek medical attention right away. The reasons people delay heading to the hospital vary: they're in denial that they might be having a heart attack; they don't want to be embarrassed should their symptoms turn out to be a "false alarm;" their symptoms aren't the obvious one—crushing chest pain radiating down the left arm; or they don't think they're at risk for a heart attack, so it's impossible they're actually having one. Or, they simply don't understand how important it is to get help quickly.

We cardiologists have a saying: "Time is muscle." The longer the delay before the blocked artery is reopened, the more heart muscle that will be damaged and the greater the risk of serious impairment or death. That's why the ER physician immediately orders an EKG and bloodwork. Typically, the EKG is performed and evaluated within about 10 minutes, and the blood is screened for *cardiac biomarkers*, which I'll talk about shortly. If evidence of a heart attack is found, the tests are repeated every three to six hours, looking for changes that help us understand the extent of injury from the heart attack.

If the EKG shows ST-segment elevation, the diagnosis is probably a STEMI, and you need to be treated right away. If there's no ST-segment elevation, your doctor then has to determine if you're having unstable angina or an NSTEMI based on the blood tests for cardiac biomarkers. If those tests are negative, you'll likely be diagnosed with either non-heart-related chest pain or unstable angina; you may be released from the emergency department and told to follow up with your cardiologist for more tests and treatment. If cardiac biomarkers are detected in your blood, you've had an NSTEMI and will need more immediate attention and treatment.

Let's take a closer look at the tests for diagnosing plumbing problems.

Electrocardiogram (EKG)

If a heart attack is a plumbing problem, why test the electrical system to diagnose it? Good question. While the parts and functions of the heart are similar in many ways to the parts and functions of a house, the systems of the heart are intimately intertwined, in ways far more sophisticated than those of a house.

The coronary arteries that provide the heart with blood run along the outside of the myocardium, the muscular walls of the heart. The electrical system runs through the walls, so if a section of the walls is being starved of oxygen, it will almost immediately affect the function of the electrical system—in this case, the heart rhythm.

If a blockage is causing a heart attack, an EKG will provide an enormous amount of information: how much muscle is damaged, how long the damage has been going on, and possibly even the location of the blocked artery. Once the information from the EKG is analyzed, we determine if additional testing is needed. If the blockage is in the back of the heart, or a small artery is blocked, a heart attack may not show up on an EKG; we then rely on blood tests.

Cardiac Biomarkers Testing

Your heart's cells require certain enzymes (proteins) to function. When your heart cells are injured, their contents (including these enzymes) are released into your bloodstream. Therefore, when we suspect a heart attack, we test the patient's blood, looking for cardiac biomarkers, or elevated levels of these enzymes.

If your cardiac biomarkers are elevated, it's an indication that your heart has been damaged—even if your EKG is normal. If your blood is positive for an enzyme called troponin, then we know we need to reopen your blocked artery to prevent more damage. *Troponin* is a protein that's released into the blood when the heart muscle is damaged. I call troponin the "drywall of your heart," because it's like the drywall in your house that can fall off the walls in a major catastrophe such as an earthquake. Typically, your doctor will order multiple blood tests over the course of a few hours to gauge any change in the biomarkers.

Echocardiogram

Doctors may also use an echocardiogram (echo), which utilizes the same technology as an ultrasound, to see your heart. (This test is described in detail in Part 4.) The echocardiogram can be very handy for doctors when it comes to diagnosing the type of heart attack a patient has had because it helps identify just how much damage has been done. Doctors call this the "degree of dysfunction." The echocardiogram can help to determine if an invasive, corrective procedure (such as bypass surgery or stenting) is urgently needed.

Angiogram (Invasive Angiography)

An *angiogram* is used to determine the extent to which your arteries are blocked. It uses X-ray imaging, but it's an invasive procedure—a very safe procedure, but a procedure nonetheless. During an angiogram, a *catheter* (a long, thin, flexible tube) is inserted into a blood vessel in your arm, groin, or neck. This tube is threaded into the arteries of your heart and releases a dye into your bloodstream. Then, X-rays are used to take pictures while the dye is moving through your heart's arteries. This procedure is also called *heart catheterization* or *cardiac catheterization* (and sometimes, just "cath"). During the angiogram, we can detect heart issues, and even repair them.

Diagnosing plumbing problems is a process that can require many tests. The EKG, cardiac biomarkers, and echocardiogram are crucial tools for diagnosing and determining the treatment for heart attack patients—whether they have unstable angina, an NSTEMI, or a STEMI.

Stress tests, coronary calcium scores, and cardiac CT angiography (CCTA) are tools for patients with stable coronary artery disease. They can detect stenosis and blockages in patients with stable angina.

CHAPTER 10

Treating Coronary Artery Disease

Remember that CAD, coronary artery disease, comes in two forms: non-obstructive and obstructive.

Non-obstructive CAD

If a patient has been diagnosed with non-obstructive CAD, the only treatment is aspirin and statins: Aspirin thins the blood, and statins calm down the plaque so it remains stable.

Aspirin

You may know someone who takes an aspirin a day to prevent blood clots. Aspirin thins the blood and reduces its ability to clot. Think about the last time you drank a milkshake through a straw. I bet it was difficult compared to drinking water. Similarly, when blood is thick, it moves very slowly through the narrowed arteries. Aspirin thins your blood and makes it less sticky, so it can more easily flow through the narrowed arteries.

Statins

I always prescribe statins for my patients with non-obstructive CAD. We've mentioned that statins are used to lower cholesterol. These drugs have also been proven to prevent plaque from growing by reducing your cholesterol levels. In addition, they can help reduce the size of plaque, and even help "calm down" inflammation within the plaque, ensuring that it will remain stable, and less prone to "volcanic eruption."

Obstructive CAD

As a reminder, obstructive coronary artery disease means that plaque has grown large enough inside your artery walls to cause a reduced flow of blood to your heart. This obstruction of blood flow then causes stable angina (predictable chest pain). Several medications can improve your symptoms, and sometimes, these medications combined with lifestyle changes may do the trick. (Since you can predict when your pain will occur, it only makes sense to stop shoveling snow, or doing whatever it is that brings on the pain.)

Medications

There are four types of drugs that can be used to manage obstructive CAD: aspirin, statins, beta blockers, and nitrates. We've talked about aspirin and statins. Let's take a look at beta blockers and nitrates.

Beta Blockers

Beta blockers help lower blood pressure and slow the heart rate, which reduces the heart's workload and its demand for oxygen. All muscles require a good supply of oxygen, and the heart is no exception: it's the hardest-working muscle in your body. It has a big job to do and requires a lot of energy. When the heart's workload is reduced, angina symptoms are prevented—or at least relieved.

Nitrates

Nitroglycerin tablets are a popular form of *nitrates* for chest pain. Nitrates dilate (open up) the arteries to the heart, which helps improve blood flow. When the flow of blood is improved, the workload on your heart is reduced, and angina is relieved.

PCI (Stenting) and Bypass Surgery

If medication and lifestyle changes don't alleviate your pain, then you may be a candidate for surgery: either *percutaneous coronary intervention* (*PCI*), which is the fancy name for *angioplasty with stenting,* or *bypass surgery,* to restore the blood flow to the heart muscle and alleviate the symptoms of stable angina. (Much more on these surgeries in the next chapter.)

These are serious procedures, and require a team of cardiologists (general and interventional cardiologists, and cardiothoracic surgeons) to determine if one of them is the best option for a patient with obstructive CAD. The patient's overall health, including kidney function, whether or not they have diabetes, and how well their heart pumps blood are all taken into consideration, along with the number, extent, and location of blockages.

CHAPTER 11

Treating Heart Attack Patients

Sirens blare and lights flash as the ambulance rushes past stopped cars and pulls into the emergency entrance of the local hospital. The EMTs rush the patient through sliding glass doors, down a long corridor, and into a brightly lit room. A surprisingly young woman appears to be having a heart attack, and medical personnel must decide on a course of treatment. Depending upon the source of her cardiac distress and the severity of her situation, they have several options from which to choose. Their decision could mean the difference between life and death.

 If you had a heart attack in the 1950s, your only treatment was weeks of bedrest! Needless to say, survival rates were low. Today, approximately 96 out of 100 heart attack patients not only survive, but are back to work in a week.[1]

Medication

Several types of drugs can prevent additional blood clots from forming in heart attack patients. There are two classes of *antithrombotics*, which you may know as blood thinners, that prevent clots from forming: *anticoagulants* and *antiplatelets*. Anticoagulants reduce the formation of fibrin, and antiplatelets prevent platelets from bonding together. Antiplatelet medications are among the most widely used drugs in the world because aspirin is an antiplatelet. Other antiplatelet drugs include dipyridamole (Persantine®), clopidogrel (Plavix®), and prasugrel (Effient®). Anticoagulants include warfarin (Coumadin®), and some newer drugs called *NOACs* (novel oral anticoagulants).

However, while these two types of drugs are preventive, they don't help us when it comes to busting up an existing clot. That's where "clot busters" (*thrombolytics*) come in. When someone is having a heart attack, we give them clot-busting medication intravenously to break up the clot, in addition to blood thinners to prevent further clotting. Examples of thrombolytic drugs used for heart attack patients include ateplase (Activase®), reteplase (Retavase®), and tenecteplase (TNKase®).

Angioplasty with Stenting

While thrombolytics used to be the primary means of treating a heart attack patient, today the preferred means of unblocking an artery—particularly in patients who are found to have ST-segment elevation—is a percutaneous coronary intervention (PCI, also known as angioplasty with stenting). As previously discussed, an angiogram or cath is used to determine the extent to which a heart attack patient's arteries are blocked. The resulting image is used to identify the location of the narrowing or blockage and determine if PCI would be effective in treating it.

Once the cardiology team has decided to proceed with a PCI, an interventional cardiologist will thread a catheter from a large artery in the groin or arm up to the patient's heart. The catheter is used to send a collapsed balloon to the blockage; the balloon is then inflated to widen the internal space in the artery, increasing the area through which blood can flow. Then, the surgeon inserts a metal mesh tube called a *coronary stent* into that same spot, expanding it against the artery walls to keep the artery open. Patients experiencing a heart attack feel instant relief as soon as the stent has been put in place.

It's critical to do this procedure quickly to restore blood flow and prevent cells in the heart's wall from dying. That's why PCI is performed in a *catheterization laboratory*, or "cath lab," a room staffed with specialists that's reserved for performing these types of interventions.

Werner Forssmann, a German physician, was the first to develop a technique for heart catheterization in 1929: He put himself under local anesthesia and inserted a catheter into a vein in his arm, putting his life at risk. He safely passed the catheter into his heart, and then walked to the X-ray department of the hospital, where a picture was taken of the catheter in his heart. In 1956, he was awarded a Nobel Prize for the development that resulted from this dangerous feat.[2]

You may hear hospitals and emergency rooms refer to "door-to-balloon" time. It's a measurement in emergency cardiac care: the amount of time between a heart attack patient's arrival at the hospital to the time they receive PCI. In the United States, hospitals cannot have a door-to-balloon time longer than 90 minutes. Door-to-balloon time has been reduced over the last decade.[3] However, hospitals and physicians can't do anything to help you if you don't call 911 and get to the hospital.

Sometimes, an artery can be blocked in more than one place at the same time. It's often possible to resolve the issue with multiple stents; however, this may not always be the best approach. Instead of unblocking an artery in multiple spots, it can be better (and less risky) to build a more permanent fix—a *coronary artery bypass.*

Coronary Artery Bypass Grafting (CABG)

Imagine the arteries of your heart as a series of interconnected highways. Near my house is Interstate 15, which runs along most of the length of Utah. If massive flooding on I-15 closed the highway for miles, traffic would be redirected to nearby highway to keep people moving to their destinations. A similar concept is used to keep blood flowing around blockages. Sometimes, when several stents are needed, we choose instead just to go around the problem areas with detours using bypass surgery. Not every patient is a candidate for coronary artery bypass surgery. Your doctor will decide based on your health, physical condition, and the extent of the damage to your plumbing.

If a highway patrol team has to fix traffic jams at every exit, they're better off diverting the traffic and using the detour route instead!

When you hear someone say they've had open heart surgery, they're referring to *coronary artery bypass surgery*, which we call CABG (pronounced like the vegetable). In this procedure, a surgeon takes veins from other parts of the patient's body to bypass multiple blockages. This creates an alternate route through which blood can flow. Since CABG is invasive, open-heart surgery, it carries with it higher immediate risks than angioplasty with stenting; but, in many cases, it provides a safer, more durable long-term solution for those with multiple blockages.

The preferred means of unblocking an artery in a heart attack patient is angioplasty with stenting. The procedure must be done quickly to restore blood flow and prevent cells in the heart's wall from dying.

CHAPTER 12

Circulation Lifestyle Tips

Now that you've learned about your heart's plumbing, you should be asking yourself: *What can I do to stay healthy?*

Start with what you put into your mouth. Your diet is often the first red flag I see when you show up in my office with plumbing blockages. Eating an unhealthy diet *can* and *does* lead to clogged plumbing. It doesn't take a genius to know you shouldn't pour grease down your kitchen sink's drain; likewise, you know that constantly stuffing fatty foods into your mouth is bad for you.

Eating healthy doesn't mean you have to give up every food you enjoy, but it does mean you need to set limits and stick to them. For example, reducing the amount of red meat you consume helps decrease the bad cholesterol in your blood. Upping the number and variety of natural fruits and vegetables you eat is also important. Three-fourths of the U.S. population is not getting the recommended daily amount of fruits and vegetables, but they are getting too much sugar, saturated fats, and sodium—thanks in large part to the over-abundance of processed foods we eat.[1] Educating yourself on healthy eating and starting the shift toward incorporating the necessary nutrients in your diet will go a long way toward a healthier heart.

Every time I think about someone who chooses to smoke knowing the potential consequences, I have to climb up on my soapbox and do a bit of preaching. You've probably heard this all your life, so let me repeat it for you one more time: Smoking increases your chances of heart-related diseases. In fact, smoking can devastate your health. It's impossible to overstate the negative health effects of tobacco. As you smoke, the nicotine and tar collect in your arteries and stay there. Tobacco smoke and nicotine almost immediately damage the blood vessels in your arteries by causing them to narrow, while plaque increases and blood pressure rises. After a widespread smoking ban in public places in various states, the states affected by the ban saw a 41% decrease in hospitalizations for heart attacks in just three years.[2] The amazing thing is that the risk factors related to smoking are completely reversible, as long as you quit—which is easier said than done. I'm sympathetic. Smoking's addictive, which is why I discourage people from ever starting.

Enough about smoking for this chapter. Let's focus on the benefits of being active. According to the President's Council on Fitness, Sports & Nutrition, more than 80% of adults in the United States don't get enough aerobic and muscle-building exercise.[3] Considering how important exercise is to your health, that's a startling number. Engaging in as little as 150 minutes of moderate physical activity a week can significantly reduce your risk for cardiovascular dysfunction. Getting enough exercise does a few things to improve your plumbing health. First, it creates good cholesterol. Typically, when we hear cholesterol, we automatically think it is bad, but good cholesterol also exists. Good cholesterol is called HDL, or high-density lipoprotein. When you have enough good cholesterol, it acts as a scavenger, searching your blood stream for bad cholesterol, fats, and plaque, and bringing them to your liver to be cleared out of your system. HDL can reduce your plaque buildup.

Exercise will also go a long way toward keeping your body at a healthy weight, which means your plumbing system doesn't have to work as hard to pump blood throughout your body. A healthy overall body weight also decreases your risk of diabetes, a condition that can be a real danger to your plumbing system, your heart health, and your body as a whole.

Recently, fish oils have been highlighted by the media as a super supplement. While it isn't always a good idea to believe the hype, in this case, it's true. EPA and DHA are dietary fats derived from fish, and they have significant health benefits. Specifically, getting enough EPA and DHA in your diet can lower your cholesterol, increase your HDL, thin your blood, reduce inflammation, stabilize plaque, and improve cellular function.

1. Eat those fruits and vegetables, which should be the bulk of your diet.
2. Quit smoking. It's never too late.
3. Exercise. You only need 150 minutes a week to start seeing the benefits.
4. Maintain a healthy weight. Extra weight and diabetes can be debilitating.

PART 4

The Myocardium: Your Heart's Walls

CHAPTER 13

How Your Myocardium Works

The *myocardium* is the muscular wall of your heart. "Heart muscle" and "heart walls" are used interchangeably, and both refer to the myocardium. Just like the walls of your home, your heart's walls provide both shelter and structure for all the other parts of your heart.

 Your heart is made almost entirely out of muscle, and if harnessed properly, it could lift over 3,000 pounds![1]

The primary function of the myocardium is to contract or squeeze to pump blood out of your heart, and then relax as your heart refills with blood. While the walls of your house don't move, they act in a similar way to support every other part of your house. They also contain important parts of the plumbing and electrical systems. When the walls of your house settle, become misaligned or are damaged, all of your doors, your plumbing, and your electrical system may be compromised; if you don't address the problem, your house may become uninhabitable. Likewise, both the plumbing and the electrical systems of the heart rest on top of the myocardium; issues with the walls of the heart can compromise these systems and vice versa.

The heart walls are thickest at the bottom of the heart (around the left and right ventricles) and are thinnest at the top (around the left and right atria). We consider the atria to be the "fillers" and the ventricles to be the "pumpers." The atria fill passively while the ventricles pump as the strong muscular walls contract and release.

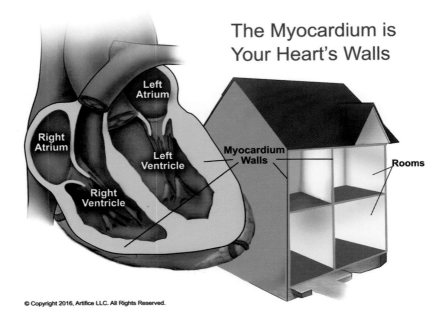

The Myocardium is Your Heart's Walls

Left Atrium

Right Atrium

Left Ventricle

Right Ventricle

Myocardium Walls

Rooms

Remember that the pumping rhythm of the heart has two phases: pump or contract (systole) and rest or expand (diastole). The heart muscle carries out these two steps thanks to prompts from the electrical system: It's triggered by an electrical signal to squeeze, followed by a pause in the signal that allows it to rest and expand.

CHAPTER 14

Myocardium Problems and Causes

Your heart's walls have a big job to do, contracting to pump blood out of the heart and then relaxing as the heart refills with returning blood. An inability to do either of these actions can negatively impact the rest of your heart.

Cardiomyopathy

Cardiomyopathy, literally "heart muscle disease," is the umbrella term for any damage or dysfunction to the walls of your heart. When your heart walls are abnormal (enlarged, thick, or rigid), it becomes harder for your heart to pump blood to the rest of your body. As cardiomyopathy gets worse, the heart becomes weaker and is no longer able to pump properly. There are different types of cardiomyopathy: Some are acquired, or developed due to another condition or disease, and others are genetic. Cardiomyopathy can lead to *congestive heart failure (CHF)*, a condition in which your heart is unable to pump blood efficiently enough to meet the body's needs. (Sometimes, "congestive heart failure" is referred to simply as "heart failure.") It can also lead to less severe dysfunction that isn't bad enough to be considered actual heart failure.

If someone mentions they suffer from congestive heart failure, a damaged heart muscle, a dilated heart or enlarged heart, they're telling you they have heart wall problems.

There are two main types of cardiomyopathy: dilated and hypertrophic. *Dilated cardiomyopathy* is a condition in which the heart's ability to pump blood is decreased because the heart's main pumping chamber, the left ventricle, is enlarged and weakened. It comes in two forms: ischemic and non-ischemic. The word *ischemia* refers to the restriction of blood supply to any organ or tissue in the body, including the heart. Like all the muscles in your body, the walls of your heart are made of oxygen-dependent cells; *ischemic cardiomyopathy* is damage to the heart's walls due to a lack of oxygen reaching the muscle. For the most part, ischemic cardiomyopathy is caused by coronary artery disease and heart attacks, both issues in the heart's plumbing: lack of blood damages the heart muscle. Ischemic cardiomyopathy is the most common cause of *systolic heart failure* or *systolic CHF.*

Non-ischemic cardiomyopathy means that the muscle is still receiving enough blood flow and oxygen, but has sustained damage from other causes. For instance, if you get a virus, it can attack and damage the heart muscle. In this case, enough blood is flowing to the heart, but the muscle is no longer strong enough to pump effectively because it's been damaged and weakened. Other causes of non-ischemic cardiomyopathy include being exposed to substances that are toxic to the heart—such as too much alcohol—or being born with an enlarged heart.

Both ischemic and non-ischemic cardiomyopathy often cause symptoms like chest pain and fatigue. This can make it hard for physicians to determine which one is affecting you until we investigate using a stress test or invasive angiogram.

Cardiomyopathy and congestive heart failure are related, but they're *not* the same thing. Cardiomyopathy refers to any condition that affects the heart walls and impairs its ability to pump normally. It can *lead* to congestive heart failure. Some people with cardiomyopathy have no signs or symptoms and need very little or no treatment; for others, the disease progresses rapidly, and the symptoms can be severe.

Congestive Heart Failure (CHF)

Not His Old Self

A week ago, Ronny had a severe heart attack caused by a blockage in one of the arteries of his heart. Luckily, he got to the ER quickly, and the doctors were able to remove the blockage. He stayed in the hospital for a few days, eating bland food and getting his vitals checked every few hours. Of course, he was happy when the nurse finally said it was time to go home. He vowed to follow all of the doctors' suggestions and clean up his lifestyle to become a new, heart-healthy man. But, a few days after going home, he felt like he still wasn't back to his old self. He was almost constantly short of breath, even when he wasn't exerting himself, and felt weak and exhausted. He'd also developed a curious and unpleasant cough. Just from knowing his recent cardiac history and hearing Ronny describe what he was feeling, I had a pretty strong suspicion that he was suffering from some degree of systolic heart failure caused by his heart attack.

When you hear the term *heart failure,* it's natural to think it means that your heart has stopped beating. Of course, if our hearts stopped beating, we'd be dead! So, heart failure doesn't mean that your heart has called it quits. It just means that it's not pumping as well as it should. This may be a bit confusing, but congestive heart failure, (again, sometimes simply called "heart failure"), isn't a heart condition. Rather, it's a symptom of ineffective pumping: When your heart isn't pumping as well as it should, it's not circulating your blood as well as it should, and that results in a buildup of fluid in your lungs and body tissues. (Think "congestion.")

Systolic Heart Failure (CHF)

Your heart muscle has a tremendous job to do: It not only pumps and fills the heart itself, but it also moves blood through your entire body. After a heart attack, the walls become weak and unable to do their job optimally, or even well enough to meet the demands of the body. This type of damage to the heart walls (ischemic cardiomyopathy) causes *systolic heart failure* because the weakness affects the pumping (systole) phase of your heartbeat. (Systolic heart failure and dilated cardiomyopathy are sometimes used synonymously.)

In a healthy heart, the left ventricle contracts fully to squeeze the blood in that ventricle out through the aorta. But, when the walls are weakened, they contract only partially, so they can expel just a fraction of the blood they would usually send out into the body. This is known as systolic heart failure, and you can imagine how it might make someone feel short of breath, weak, and tired. Other symptoms of systolic heart failure include excess fluid around the lungs (*pleural effusion*), and in the lungs (*pulmonary edema*).

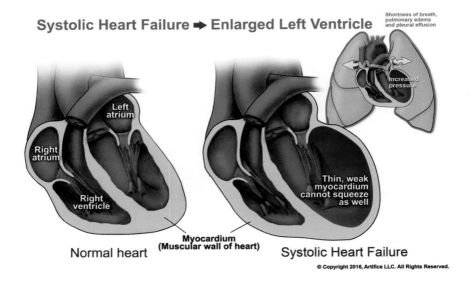

Systolic Heart Failure ➡ Enlarged Left Ventricle

Shortness of breath, pulmonary edema and pleural effusion

Left atrium

Right atrium

Right ventricle

Increased pressure

Thin, weak myocardium cannot squeeze as well

Myocardium (Muscular wall of heart)

Normal heart   Systolic Heart Failure

© Copyright 2016, Artifice LLC. All Rights Reserved.

Heart Attacks as a Cause of Systolic Heart Failure (Dilated Cardiomyopathy)

Ischemic cardiomyopathy is the most common form of dilated cardiomyopathy. It occurs when the heart is deprived of oxygen due to a heart attack or blockage in its plumbing system (arteries). If the plumbing gets blocked on one side of the heart, then the corresponding wall can sustain damage. However, if there are multiple plumbing blockages throughout the left and right side of the heart, then all of the walls suffer.

If someone suffering from a heart attack reaches the ER in time, and their arteries can be opened, then the heart walls suffer little or no damage, and the heart attack is considered a "small" one. But, if blood flow isn't restored quickly, part of the heart muscle begins to die, and the attack is deemed a "large" one.

Imagine you had a plumbing leak behind the walls of your home in which water gushed out of the pipes, soaking the surrounding areas and causing significant damage. You'd rush to call a plumber so he could repair the leak, but after he'd packed up his equipment and given you your bill, you'd still be left with a huge mess to clean up. Your walls may have become warped, moldy, sunken, or expanded, depending on how much water was present, and how far it spread. The same applies to the walls in your heart after a heart attack: It leaves damage behind, depending on how quickly the issue was resolved.

Ischemic injury to the heart impacts the entire body: Since the heart isn't able to effectively propel blood throughout the body, the blood isn't able to carry nutrients to where they're needed or adequately remove waste products.

Many people think that if they survive a heart attack, they've dodged the bullet and get to go on with life, albeit with making some changes in their habits. Unfortunately, that's not always true. Once muscle tissue is deprived of oxygen, the damage may not be reversible. Each time this happens—as in the case of someone who has multiple heart attacks—the walls are damaged and weakened even more. Here's the ironic part: as we've gotten better and better at treating heart attacks and keeping people who have them alive, the number of patients with heart failure is increasing. While more and more patients who suffer heart attacks survive, we often can't undo the damage.

Infectious Causes of Systolic Heart Failure (Dilated Cardiomyopathy)

Myocarditis, an inflammation of the heart walls (the myocardium), is the most common cause of non-ischemic cardiomyopathy: The heart muscle is damaged and weakened by a virus, though the heart's plumbing is normal. The most common cause of myocarditis is a viral infection caused by certain viruses, fungi, bacteria, or parasites. Myocarditis is something all cardiologists hate to see. Most often the patient is young and getting myocarditis isn't their fault. They did everything right … they were just unlucky.

Myocarditis produces the same symptoms as other causes of systolic heart failure: chest pain, shortness of breath, and fatigue. But, it differs from other causes in that the blood vessels (the pipes) are clear; instead, the myocardium itself is infected and unable to function properly. In fact, myocarditis can appear very similar to a heart attack, and sometimes doctors need to use magnetic resonance imaging of the heart (or cardiac MRI) to determine which condition a patient is experiencing.

Other Causes of Systolic Heart Failure (Dilated Cardiomyopathy)

Plumbing problems aren't the only thing that can cause damage to the walls of your home; likewise, a heart attack isn't the only cause of dilated cardiomyopathy or systolic heart failure. Several substances are toxic to your heart walls, including illegal drugs like cocaine, but also some anticancer drugs used in chemotherapy. Unfortunately, some people who survive cancer die from heart disease caused by chemotherapy. Others sustain heart damage from radiation used to treat breast and other cancers.

Any toxin you put into your body can cause heart damage although, luckily, most don't. Stimulants—such as amphetamines, and even some drugs used to treat attention deficit hyperactivity disorder (ADHD)—can cause the heart to spasm and the arteries to constrict. While this is not an actual heart attack, the symptoms and side effects are the same as those of heart attack. Like a kink in a garden hose that hinders or stops the flow of water, stimulants cause the arteries to constrict or tighten, dramatically reducing the flow of blood, which is another cause of ischemia.

Virtually the only treatment for heart failure at the beginning of the 1950s was the use of mercury-containing diuretics that were typically given intravenously. (We now know that mercury can be toxic to the human body.) In the latter part of that decade the arrival of new drugs for the treatment of fluid retention—such as chloro-thiazide and spironolactone—transformed the way heart failure is managed.[1]

Broken Heart Syndrome

While there are many types of non-ischemic dilated cardiomyopathy (heart muscle disease), one of the most interesting is known as *broken heart syndrome.*

When patients arrive at the ER with symptoms of heart failure but show no signs of blocked arteries, we say they have broken heart syndrome or *Takotsubo cardiomyopathy.* Technically, it's a heart attack; but it's caused by stress or a virus, and not a plumbing blockage. It's only in the last 10 years that this disease has become widely known and understood. Old movies used to depict a character clutching his chest and collapsing with a heart attack after hearing some shocking and terrible news. Back then, cardiologists *knew* a heart attack didn't work like that. Hearts attacks couldn't be brought on by stress or shock—that only happened in the movies! But in 1990, this belief began to crumble when Japan officially recognized the first case of Takotsubo cardiomyopathy. It took until 1998 for the United States to accept the diagnosis, and since then, interest, attention, and research have increased exponentially.

Takotsubo cardiomyopathy is the abrupt onset of symptoms related to heart wall damage. It occurs during or directly after high levels of stress and looks very much like an ordinary heart attack caused by clogged arteries. Broken heart syndrome creates an abnormal electrocardiogram (EKG) and high levels of biomarkers. It's not until an angiogram has been performed that the doctor can see the arteries aren't blocked and can distinguish between the two diagnoses. (In rare cases, a physician may detect blocked arteries in a patient with Takotsubo cardiomyopathy as it's possible for stress to cause arteries to spasm, which then leads to a blockage. But, that's the exception rather than the norm.)

When a patient's blood is tested during a Takotsubo cardiomyopathy, it shows very high levels of adrenaline. And, it's well-known that the sudden onset of excessive stress or continuous stress over time causes a massive release of adrenaline. There's no coincidence here: While some amount of stress can be a positive force in our lives, too much stress is detrimental, not only to our mental health but also to our hearts.

Alcoholic Cardiomyopathy

Alcohol is a good-news, bad-news proposition when it comes to your heart: While limited alcohol use can help to clean out your heart's plumbing system, drinking too much can be toxic. Alchohol abuse can lead to wall problems (dilated cardiomyopathy and congestive heart failure), as well as problems with your heart's rhythm. Alcoholic cardiomyopathy causes one-third of all cases of non-ischemic dilated cardiomyopathy in the United States.[2]

Women should limit themselves to one drink per day
and men should limit themselves to two daily drinks.

Diastolic Heart Failure (CHF)

When you have systolic heart failure (a weak heart muscle), your heart can't pump effectively, but in *diastolic heart failure*, the problem has nothing to do with the function of the pump. In fact, your ventricles (pumpers) work quite well. When you have diastolic heart failure, your heart can't *fill* adequately due to a stiffening of the heart muscle. The primary problem is that the ventricles (pumpers) aren't able to effectively fill with blood from the atria (fillers) because the muscle tissue doesn't relax when it should. So, the left ventricle pumps the blood adequately, but then struggles during the diastole (the resting phase), and isn't able to fill properly. A stiff, engorged heart muscle doesn't allow enough blood to enter the ventricles during rest. As a result, it can't pump enough blood out through the aorta to the body during the pumping phase—and the blood may even go backward and end up in your lungs—leading to heart failure symptoms such as shortness of breath and fatigue. Diastolic dysfunction usually refers to reduced performance of the left ventricle, but sometimes both ventricles are affected.

***Your heart is a pump, working against the pressure of the rest of your body.
If the heart has to work harder than it normally would,
it becomes stiff and thick, and can't function properly.***

Imagine how you'd feel if you were never able to rest. Eventually, you'd find yourself mentally and physically exhausted, unable to put in enough effort to perform even small tasks well. We use our weekends and vacations to recharge. The same applies to the heart. It works hard day after day and needs times of rest to refill. The resting phase of the heart is vital to its proper function, just as good, solid rest is crucial to our overall well-being.

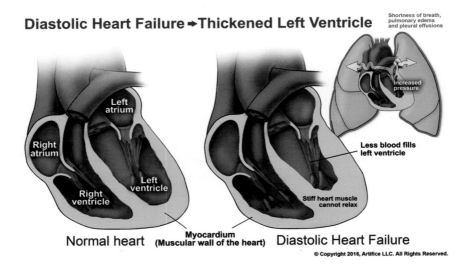

Diastolic Heart Failure ➡ Thickened Left Ventricle
Shortness of breath, pulmonary edema and pleural effusions

Left atrium
Right atrium
Left ventricle
Right ventricle
Increased pressure
Less blood fills left ventricle
Stiff heart muscle cannot relax

Normal heart   Myocardium (Muscular wall of the heart)   Diastolic Heart Failure

When you return to the gym after an extended absence, you may find yourself sore and stiff the next morning. Simply walking up and down the stairs may be difficult until your muscles have recovered. This is very similar to what happens in your heart during diastolic dysfunction. Your heart may look stronger, but we know that it has become less effective rather than more effective. The muscle itself isn't damaged; it's just been worked too hard. Like your bicep after too many dumbbell lifts, your heart becomes stronger and beefed up when it's worked too hard for too long, causing the muscle to become stiff and less elastic.

The heart does the most physical work of any muscle during a lifetime.[3]

Causes of Diastolic Heart Failure

It's important to keep your blood pressure in check. High blood pressure, also called hypertension, is the most common cause of a stiff heart muscle. This is called *hypertensive heart disease.* You may wonder how high blood pressure can cause a stiffening of your heart muscle. When your heart pumps, it's pumping against the pressure from the rest of the body, (your blood pressure). If your blood pressure is too high, your heart has to work harder each time it beats to overcome that pressure and deliver blood throughout your body. So, your heart muscle becomes stiff and thickened, not from working out too much at the gym, but rather from trying to pump against this high blood pressure a million times a day! That's how high blood pressure or hypertension becomes the leading cause of diastolic heart failure—and why it's so important to keep your blood pressure down.

The second most common cause is aging: The heart has been pumping for so long that it no longer functions as well as it used to. Think about it: If your house has been standing for 70 or 80 years, natural wear and tear will begin to show on its walls. And, if you were working any other muscle continuously every single day of your life, you might start to notice that it's not performing as it once did—just like your bicep fatigues if you work it too hard and for too long.

In addition to high blood pressure and aging, there are also genetic causes of diastolic heart failure, including hypertrophic cardiomyopathy, which I'll talk about in just a moment.

To keep the two types of heart failure straight, think of systolic as weak and diastolic as stiff. A weak muscle can't squeeze effectively while a thick muscle can't rest well enough to let the rooms of the heart refill.

Hypertrophic Cardiomyopathy (HCM)

Some people are born with genes that cause the walls of their hearts to thicken. For this reason, the term cardiomyopathy not only applies to conditions causing damaged heart muscle; it also refers to conditions causing a thick dysfunctional heart muscle.

Known as *hypertrophic cardiomyopathy* (HCM), this genetically induced thickening of the heart walls can cause sudden death during exercise and is the number one cause of death among athletes. The walls of the heart become so thick that they decrease the size of the heart's rooms, so they can't hold or pump as much blood. Although these thick walls appear strong, they're dysfunctional. We'll talk about your heart's electrical system in Part 5, but for now, just be aware that the electrical system in your heart's walls can become scarred, putting patients at risk for abnormal heart rhythm and even sudden death. Some people with HCM have no symptoms at all and live normal lives. Others may experience symptoms such as shortness of breath, and may need to limit their exercise to moderate-intensity activities.

In the case of the hypertrophic cardiomyopathy and any other genetic cardiomyopathies, your doctor will likely suggest screening family members, even those who have no symptoms, for heart issues. It's better to spot and treat a family member who might have the same problem before they begin to experience symptoms, to prevent irreversible damage to the heart.

Cardiomyopathy means physical damage or dysfunction to the walls of your heart. Cardiomyopathy with a damaged muscle is called dilated cardiomyopathy; in patients with a thick heart muscle, it's called hypertrophic cardiomyopathy. Dilated cardiomyopathy can be ischemic (not enough blood flow or oxygen) or non-ischemic (some outside factor is doing a number on the heart's walls). This damage can come from causes you acquired or were born with. The result is a weak (damaged) or thick (dysfunctional) heart wall.

Congestive heart failure is a symptom of ineffective pumping. When your heart isn't pumping as well as it should, it's not circulating your blood as well as it should, and that results in a buildup of fluid in your lungs and body tissues. (Think "congestion.")

CHAPTER 15

Diagnosing Myocardium Problems

The initial procedure for diagnosing heart wall problems is similar to the process for identifying other types of heart issues: We begin with a medical history and a physical exam.

My stethoscope often provides me with some useful information: I listen for a rapid heartbeat, which means the heart has lost some power and is trying to make up for it by beating faster. I may also hear crackling sounds and heart murmurs, which suggest an issue with the myocardium (heart walls). These crackles are signs of water collecting in your lungs, and the murmurs are from the backflow of the blood through the mitral valve into the lungs. I also check the patient's ankles, feet, legs, and abdomen looking for any swelling or bloating, signs of fluid buildup—a result of poor right ventricular function.

In most cases, I order the same diagnostic tests: an EKG, echo, chest X-rays, and bloodwork. Let's look at how some specific tests can provide clues regarding the state of your heart's walls.

Electrocardiogram

Remember that a normal EKG suggests there's nothing critically wrong with the heart muscle. In patients with heart failure, however, we tend to see variations from a normal EKG reading. It's also possible to detect a thickening of the wall of the left ventricle (known as *left ventricular hypertrophy*) or a stretching or thinning of that ventricle (*left ventricular dilatation*) on an EKG.

Chest X-Ray

A chest X-ray can allow your doctor to see if you have an enlarged heart, and spot other telltale signs of heart wall problems. This test can also help your doctor determine how advanced your condition is. For example, if you're in an early state of heart failure, an X-ray might reveal enlarged blood vessels in your chest. But, if you're already in a more advanced stage, an X-ray could show that you have pulmonary edema (fluid in your lungs), and pleural effusion (excess fluid around the lungs).

Bloodwork

Several blood tests can provide clues about how your heart is functioning, as well as what may be causing any heart wall problems. These tests include:

- CBC (complete blood count), which can reveal that you have anemia or an infection—both of which can cause heart failure.
- CMP (comprehensive metabolic profile), which indicates how well certain organs (such as your liver and kidneys) are functioning as they can also get damaged in patients with severe heart failure.
- Thyroid Profile (TSH, FT3, and FT4), which can reveal if thyroid issues are leading to problems with your heart's walls. Both low and high thyroid levels can cause congestive heart failure and cardiomyopathy.
- BNP (B-type natriuretic peptide) test, which measures the level of a hormone that rises when you have heart failure. We use this test to help us gauge the amount of excess fluid in your body.

Echocardiogram

Often the most telling tests cardiologists conduct on patients who might have heart failure is the echocardiogram. The ultrasound waves create a moving picture of your heart walls and how they function in real time. The echo helps your doctor determine the severity of your heart failure, and whether it's due to systolic or diastolic dysfunction. An echocardiogram can also reveal places where your heart might be thicker or thinner than normal.

Combining the echo with a stress test (known as "stress echocardiography") allows us to diagnose heart wall issues with greater accuracy. By pairing these tests, we can see if you have areas of decreased blood flow to the myocardium in response to exercise, which might indicate ischemic damage caused by coronary artery disease. While an echocardiogram can be used to detect heart wall abnormalities, to best gauge how efficiently the heart is pumping, doctors use the echo to measure something called the *left ventricular ejection fraction*, or just *ejection fraction (EF)*.

Stress Test

Many heart issues, such as an irregular heartbeat, aren't apparent on the EKG during rest. The stress test is crucial in diagnosing the cause of heart failure. As I've explained, ischemic cardiomyopathy is caused by a lack of blood flow, while non-ischemic cardiomyopathy is damage to the heart by some other means. A stress test is the one crucial diagnostic tool that allows us to determine the difference: If the results show no signs of a plumbing blockage (ischemia), your cardiomyopathy is probably non-ischemic: Ischemic cardiomyopathy caused by coronary artery disease and plumbing blockage can be easily picked up by an abnormal stress test.

Ejection Fraction: Measuring the Severity of Systolic Heart Failure

If you have weak heart walls, the volume of blood your heart pumps in one minute (*cardiac output*) is decreased, and your heart doesn't push out as much blood as it should to the rest of the body. *Ejection fraction (EF)* is an important measurement that determines the amount of blood leaving your heart with each pump. This measurement is your *ejection fraction score*. A typical, healthy score is about 60%, which means 60% of the blood in your ventricle is leaving each time, and about 40% remains in the ventricle for your heart to use.

When I say "ejection fraction," many patients hear "ejection fracture." It makes sense since a fracture indicates damage and they understand that something in the heart is broken. But EF is a diagnostic measurement, not a state of damage. It's the most important measure of the severity of systolic heart failure or dysfunction, so it's important to understand.

During an echocardiogram, an echocardiographer calculates your heart's ability to pump blood from the left ventricle to the body. Remember, your heart works in two phases, resting and pumping. During rest, the ventricle fills with blood, and during pumping, it sends out blood. When the ventricle rests, it should fill to 100% capacity with blood. However, when the ventricle contracts and pumps blood to the rest of your body, it should only push out about 60% of the blood it's holding. The heart needs to keep some blood to function properly.

The devil is in the details! Depending on the type of test used to measure your ejection fraction, and the technician performing the test, your results will be different.

Your ejection fraction score shows your doctor the extent of your heart wall failure and allows your health care team to develop the best possible treatment. An ejection fraction score below 60% means your heart may be weak. It may also mean that your arteries are blocked. An ejection fraction score between 55% and 70% is usually considered normal, while values between 40% and 55% are considered borderline. A borderline score indicates that you may have a weak heart, but the situation isn't considered critical. A score below 40%, however, is seen as dangerous and immediate action is needed. (Please note that the cutoff points for what's considered normal and critical vary somewhat depending on which guidelines your cardiologist is using.)

Severity of Systolic Heart Failure or Dilated Cardiomyopathy

Ejection Fraction Score	What it Means
55-70%	Normal ejection fraction. The echocardiogram report would state that your heart function is normal.
40-55%	Below normal, borderline ejection fraction. The echocardiogram report would state, "Mild left ventricle (LV) dysfunction."
35-40%	Moderately low ejection fraction, moderate heart failure. The echocardiogram report would state, "Moderate left ventricle (LV) dysfunction or cardiomyopathy."
<35%	Severely low ejection fraction, severe heart failure. The echocardiogram report would state, "Severe left ventricle (LV) dysfunction or cardiomyopathy." The patient may be at risk for life-threatening irregular heart rhythms.

A lot of people think ejection fraction is an exact measurement and that any small variation is meaningful. Unfortunately, this misunderstanding can cause unnecessary worry. During an echo, the sonographer (the technician performing the test) views a 2-D image of your heart on a monitor and then traces around the area to be measured. Then, a computer uses this tracing to calculate your ejection fraction score. Since no two sonographers are going to trace the same area the same way, you may receive slightly differing scores depending on the person who performed the test.

Your EF can also be measured during other tests such as a nuclear stress test, cardiac catheterization, MRI (magnetic resonance imaging), or CT (computerized tomography). However, these methods are less common, and different techniques may result in a slightly different score than you'd receive if the test were performed via an echo. The bottom line is that you shouldn't worry about a bit of discrepancy between your EF scores. Although your ejection fraction score is important and it's certainly best when it doesn't go down, don't get too fixated on your EF number.

CHAPTER 16

Treating Myocardium Problems

Treatment for the walls of the heart isn't always aggressive and is never a quick fix. When patients hear diagnoses like cardiomyopathy and congestive heart failure, they get scared and just want a surgeon to come in and fix it. Unfortunately, however, that's usually not possible when it comes to wall problems.

There are three main goals when treating cardiomyopathy:

1. Manage the cause.
2. Minimize the symptoms.
3. Stop the progression and help the recover heart function.

Congestive heart failure can sometimes "flare up" and come on suddenly, a condition we call *acute heart failure* or *decompensated heart failure*. When that happens, you usually need to be hospitalized to get your symptoms under control. Heart failure is the number one cause of hospitalization among patients older than 65.[1]

Managing the Cause

When you have a thick-walled heart, your doctor will first try to address the issue by reducing whatever it was that stressed the myocardium in the first place. So, if your cardiomyopathy has been caused by a blocked artery or high blood pressure, unblocking that artery and lowering your blood pressure may be enough to allow the heart to recover. Also, your doctor may suggest lifestyle changes, including quitting smoking, losing excess weight, better managing your stress, and avoiding the use of alcohol and illegal drugs. Over time, your heart wall may begin to heal, allowing it to function in a healthier fashion, a process we call *reverse remodeling*. Even if your cardiomyopathy has a genetic basis, reducing things that stress the heart may help you live longer and with fewer symptoms.

The way to treat a thick-walled heart is by reducing the stress on the heart itself.

In addition to these strategies that address the source of stress on the walls of your heart, there are devices and surgeries that can be used to treat cardiomyopathy.

Minimizing the Symptoms of Congestive Heart Failure

Remember that congestive heart failure occurs when your heart doesn't pump blood as well as it should. Since patients who have heart failure often have other chronic conditions such as lung disease, diabetes, and renal (kidney) disease, heart failure treatment often has to be modified to accommodate the treatment of other diseases and conditions. My Artisan's Approach™ comes into play here. When a patient comes to see me, I can't consider just one part of their health, just as I can't read one chapter of a book and get the most out of it. As an artisan, I look at how any treatment I prescribe might affect—or be affected by—everything else that's taking place in a patient's body. I need to understand the overall picture.

Congestive heart failure gets worse over time. A primary goal of heart failure treatment is slowing the progression of the disease. Guidelines for treating heart failure are extensive and well-studied pathways for treatment. However, even within them, there's a need for a tailored approach. We, the physicians, need to see you on a regular basis, monitor your kidney function, and slowly adjust your medications, so they best address your condition. While the guidelines provide a valuable basis for your treatment plan, we need to consider your unique case and involve you in making decisions for you to get top-notch care. All of the treatment strategies mentioned in this chapter are most effective when they're part of a customized plan that you and your doctor develop together.

The Congestive Heart Failure "Cocktail"

"Doc," says George as he sits in my examining room and I listen to his heartbeat, "I hate taking medicine, and having to take three pills at one time is just too much. Can't we do away with a couple of them?"

"Well, we can," I reply, "but just taking one pill—or even two—won't do you any good. Do you want to get better?"

After being diagnosed with congestive heart failure, many patients complain that the doctor puts them on too many pills. What they may not understand is that each pill has an additive effect on their overall health and recovery. We're not trying to make it difficult for patients! Through research, we've found there's a "cocktail" of heart pills, each with a different purpose. If you don't take them in the right combination, you'll miss out on the best treatment. Each pill targets a different symptom or treats the heart failure itself.

The medications your doctor may prescribe to help your heart recover are divided into four classes: diuretics, ACE Inhibitors and ARBs, beta blockers, and aldosterone antagonists. Diuretics primarily serve to flush the excess water from your system so you can breathe better, helping to meet the first goal of treatment: managing symptoms. ACE Inhibitors, beta blockers, and aldosterone antagonists address symptoms as well, but also help your heart recover function and prevent your condition from progressing. Research shows that these three classes of drugs work together to help your heart recover; so, we use all three when it's possible to give you the best shot at improving your heart function. All drug treatments will be closely monitored by your doctor to make sure you're taking the medicine that's right for you, in a dose that's effective.

Please don't stop taking your medicine.

Failure to take medication as prescribed is one of the leading causes of acute heart failure. Sometimes patients stop taking their medications for financial reasons; sometimes they just forget. Other times, they think their medications are to blame for side effects they're feeling; but, instead of investigating the issue with their doctors, they try stopping the drugs themselves to see if their side effects disappear. To be fair, there are other causes of acute heart failure, but please don't stop taking your prescriptions without consulting with your physician. If you don't take your medications, you'll miss out on the best possible treatment for your condition.

Diuretics

Diuretics are essential in minimizing symptoms. Often referred to as "water pills," they're recommended to get rid of fluid in the lungs, legs, and belly in heart failure patients who are retaining water. There are three types of diuretics (thiazide, loop, and potassium-sparing diuretics), each of which affects a different part of your kidneys. The type of diuretic prescribed depends on the condition being treated. A few common diuretics are hydrochlorothiazide (HCTZ®), furosemide (Lasix®), bumetanide (Bumex®), and torsemide (Demadex®). Torsemide is the newest and most easily absorbed.

The three remaining classes of drugs are used only for patients with systolic heart failure, as they don't benefit patients with diastolic heart failure.

These three categories of drugs have not only been shown to prevent progression of the disease and improve ejection fraction, but they also help patients with systolic heart failure live longer.

Angiotensin-converting-enzyme (ACE) inhibitors, beta blockers, and aldosterone antagonists all help the heart muscle regain its function and reverse remodel the ventricle. In addition, these three classes of drugs help to control blood pressure.

ACE Inhibitors (ACEI)

Angiotensin-converting enzyme (ACE) inhibitors help relax and open your blood vessels. They do this by blocking the production of an enzyme in your body called angiotensin II, which narrows your blood vessels and causes your heart to work harder to pump blood. We recommend them for patients with dilated cardiomyopathy or systolic heart failure. ACE inhibitor drugs all end with the suffix -pril; examples include enalapril (Vasotec®), captopril (Capoten®), lisinopril (Zestril®), and ramipril (Altace®). In addition to minimizing symptoms, this group of drugs helps to prevent the disease from progressing and lowers your risk of heart-related problems and death. (We doctors call this "improving survival or longevity.") ACE inhibitors are used to control blood pressure in patients with diastolic heart failure.

Angiotensin Receptor Blockers (ARB)

A patient who can't take an ACE inhibitor because of the side effects (usually an annoying dry cough) might be prescribed an angiotensin receptor blocker (ARB). These drugs, which include losartan (Cozaar®) and valsartan (Diovan®), have many of the same benefits as ACE inhibitors. However, ACE inhibitors are more effective in treating heart failure.

> *If you have a dry cough and doctors can't pinpoint the cause, look at your list of medications. If you're taking an ACE inhibitor, bring it to our doctor's attention. Switching to another medication may halt your hacking.*

Beta Blockers (BB)

Like ACE inhibitors, beta blockers both reduce symptoms and improve longevity in systolic heart failure or dilated cardiomyopathy patients. These drugs slow your heart rate and lower your blood pressure, which can help repair cellular damage to the myocardium, allowing your heart to heal. All drugs belonging to this class of medications end with the suffix -olol. Common beta blockers include metoprolol (Lopressor® and Toprol-XL®), carvedilol (Coreg®), atenolol

(Tenormin®), bisoprolol (Zebeta®), nadolol (Corgard®), and propranolol (Inderal LA®, InnoPran XL®). Only three beta blockers have shown a clear-cut benefit in reducing death rates and improving survival: bisoprolol, carvedilol, and sustained release metoprolol (Toprol-XL®). The others can still be used in patients with diastolic heart failure to reduce blood pressure.

Aldosterone Antagonists (AA)

Diuretics can control symptoms, but they don't help to heal the heart muscle. But, a class of diuretics known as *aldosterone antagonists* help repair the heart and improve left ventricular function. In addition to minimizing symptoms, they prevent heart failure from progressing, ultimately lowering the risk of death from heart-related problems.

Mechanical Support

When your heart has become so damaged that it can no longer pump blood well enough to keep you alive, it's time for a more mechanical option (*mechanical circulatory support*). We use many devices, such as *biventricular pacemakers* to help your heart pump and prevent life-threatening rhythm problems. (A *pacemaker* is a battery-powered device that's surgically implanted under the skin to help the heart beat in a more balanced way.)

Let's take a look at several mechanical options available to help those with severe heart failure.

Cardiac Resynchronization Therapy (CRT)

A specialized type of pacemaker, the *cardiac resynchronization therapy (CRT) device* is designed to resynchronize the beats of your heart, help reduce the size of the left ventricle, and assist in improving its ability to pump. In patients with systolic heart failure, we don't use a CRT device to compensate for lack of power (what I call "electricity"), but rather to stimulate the heart muscle in a particular pattern to help it pump more efficiently. As your general contractor, I work in close collaboration with my electrician colleague to select the patients that are the best candidates. Sometimes I use the results of an echocardiogram to make this decision. At the heart of my Artisan's Approach™ is the fact that not all patients with heart failure are the same.

Ventricular Assist Device (VAD) or Artificial Heart

Recently, we've started to use artificial pumps, which are surgically implanted and can take over for a failed ventricle. The *ventricular assist device* (VAD) is a real wonder of medical technology. The VAD is a mechanical pump that takes over for your heart to relieve severe symptoms of heart failure and keep you alive. We mostly use VADs for patients recovering from surgery, to temporarily decrease the heart's workload and give it a chance to recover until their heart heal from the damage with appropriate time and medicines.

One of the primary purposes of VADs is to "bridge" a patient (i.e., keep them alive) until they're able to receive a heart transplant. This was the case for former Vice President Dick Cheney, who received an LVAD (left ventricular assist advice) after suffering five heart attacks. This device kept his heart beating for 20 months until he received a heart transplant.

One of the wonders of this technology is that in some patients, just giving the left ventricle a break from pumping blood to the entire body enables the ventricle to heal and recover its natural function—or, at least enough of it that the patient can delay and sometimes avoid a heart transplant. However, please understand that this is rare. Still, because VADs have been so effective at what they do, some patients get an implanted VAD (there are external devices too) instead of a heart transplant. They just live with the mechanical assist for the rest of their lives.

Cardiac Transplant

Sometimes, if your house is damaged beyond repair, the only option might be to tear it down and build a new house. That's obviously not possible when it comes to your heart, but a heart transplant is possible.

If the disease has progressed to the point of no repair, a team of doctors opts for a heart transplant. The patient's failing heart is removed and replaced with a healthy heart from a deceased donor. Although transplants are considered the only available *cure* for heart failure, they're the last resort and performed only on patients who are in the final stages of heart failure. A patient is a good candidate for a heart transplant if they're in advanced heart failure, but otherwise healthy. So, patients with other complications such as liver damage, cancer, or lung disease might not be eligible for a transplant. Similarly, patients struggling with drug or alcohol addiction aren't quality candidates for a heart transplant.

Dr. Robert Jarvik is known as the inventor of the first successful permanent artificial heart, the Jarvik 7. It was successfully implanted in a human in 1982.[2]

CHAPTER 17

Myocardium Lifestyle Tips

I've talked about food before, and I'm about to talk about it again. What you put in your body matters to your overall health and your heart health. Beyond adding fruits and veggies to your diet and limiting your red meat, you have to start being mindful of the sodium you're taking in. Sodium isn't just found in a salt shaker. It hides in almost all of our prepackaged foods. Even foods that claim to be "natural" and "healthy" are sometimes secretly loaded with sodium. It's estimated that 75% of American's sodium comes from processed foods rather than table salt.[1] Sodium can cause you to retain more water, making it harder for your heart to pump against the increased fluid. It can also lead to high blood pressure, which as you now know can lead to heart failure.

One slice of American cheese has 443 mg of sodium. One cup of canned soup can have almost your entire daily allotment of sodium. This leads me to my next tip. Read the labels. It's nobody's responsibility but your own to make sure the food you eat is right for you. Keep in mind that labels can be deceiving. For a food to be labeled "low sodium" it cannot exceed 140 mg per serving, while a package labeled "no sodium" cannot exceed 5 mg of sodium per serving. But, beware: Just because a package says "unsalted" doesn't mean that it's sodium-free. Be a savvy consumer.

Manage your stress to avoid stress-induced cardiomyopathy. We don't live in bubbles and it's not possible to avoid stress entirely. But, you can manage your stress: Meditation, yoga, taking the time to unwind each day, exercising, listening to music, and having a good belly laugh are all ways to reduce stress.

Most doctors and nutritionists tell you to drink a lot of fluids each day, so the advice I'm about to give you will seem both contradictory and counterintuitive. When you have a history of heart failure, your heart doesn't pump out enough blood. This, along with too much sodium, can cause excess fluid to build up in your body, putting too much strain on your heart. The solution is often a diuretic pill. When that pill isn't enough, I ask my heart failure patients to limit their fluid intake to only two liters a day. Reducing liquids and limiting sodium will help flush your system of excess water and make it easier for your heart to work properly. But of course, always check with your cardiologist.

1. Ease off the sodium: Consume no more than 2,000 milligrams a day.
2. Read your food labels: Don't get tricked into eating the things you're trying to avoid.
3. Take your prescribed medicine: You have it for a reason.
4. If you have heart failure, limit your fluids and give your heart a rest.

PART 5

The Rhythm: Your Heart's Electrical System

CHAPTER 18

How Your Heart's Rhythm Works

When you wake up in the middle of the night and turn on the lamp beside your bed, the room fills with light. This is thanks to the electrical current coming from the power lines outside your home, in through the breaker panel, and traveling through wires that run throughout your home. The wires that transmit this current are hidden in your walls, but power all of your outlets, lights, and appliances—just waiting to deliver electricity where and when you need it. A very similar system is found in your heart, except that you *always* need it.

You've probably heard, or personally used, "heartbeat" expressions hundreds of times throughout the years: "It was over in a heartbeat." "I'll be there in a heartbeat." "Life can change in a heartbeat." But what, exactly, is a heartbeat? It's a single cycle—controlled by the electrical system of the heart—during which your heart's chambers relax and contract to circulate blood, as the valves between the chambers open and close to allow the continual flow of blood. Your heart's electrical system is responsible for creating the signals that tell your heart to beat.

 This complex series of events that make up a heartbeat happens 60 to 90 times a minute, 60 minutes an hour, 24 hours a day without any conscious effort from you. That's about 2.5 billion times in a lifetime—and you're hardly even aware that it's happening!

Electricity is a wonderful thing, powering just about everything in our homes. We forget how much we rely on electrical power—until it goes out and we're inconvenienced: We can't turn on the lights, the television, or a hairdryer. The air conditioning stops blowing cold air and the oven won't work. We get frustrated knowing there's not a thing we can do, except wait until the power is restored, and then all will run smoothly once again. But when a power outage occurs in your heart, rather than suffering a minor annoying inconvenience that will eventually be corrected, you could be out of luck. When you have no power in your heart, none of the other systems can do their jobs: The walls won't contract, the valves won't open and close, and the blood won't flow. Obviously, this is something you want to avoid at all costs because an extended power outage in the heart can mean death. Just as most of our homes have no backup generators, neither does your heart. You only have one electrical system, and it certainly pays to keep it in top working order at all times.

If you've ever had electrical work done in your house, you can appreciate the intricate network of wires that stretch behind the walls of your home. The wiring for something as simple as an overhead light appears complicated to anyone who's unfamiliar with electrical work. Your heart's electrical system may seem similarly complicated if you're unschooled in cardiology. Six interconnected parts tell the heart when to contract:

1. *Sinoatrial (SA) node*
2. *Atrioventricular (AV) node*
3. *Bundle of His*
4. *Right bundle branch (RBB)*
5. *Left bundle branch (LBB)*
6. *Purkinje or ventricular fibers*

Your brain signals the heart's *sinoatrial (SA) node,* located in the right atrium, to generate an electrical impulse, which starts the heartbeat. The signal travels through pathways, like wires in your house, and spreads through the left and right atria (the two upper chambers), triggering them to contract. The electrical signal then moves to the *atrioventricular (AV) node*—located between the atria and the ventricles—and continues through the *bundle of His.* This bundle branches into yet more "wires" that extend around the left and right ventricles, aptly called the left and right bundle branches. The signal goes out to the muscle fibers of the ventricles through the Purkinje fibers, which are the final "thin wires" that spread the signal through the muscle fibers of the ventricles. Finally, the ventricles relax, and the process starts again in the SA node.

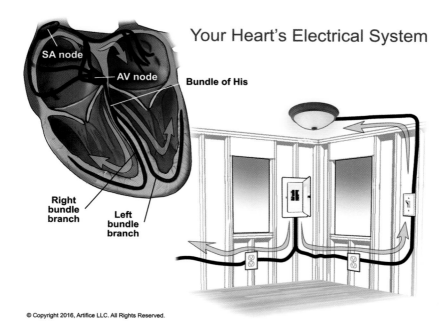

Your Heart's Electrical System

SA node

AV node

Bundle of His

Right bundle branch

Left bundle branch

The SA node, sometimes referred to as the *sinus node,* is the "natural pacemaker" of the heart. It's simply a cluster of specialized cells. Because of its origin, the natural rhythm of the heartbeat is called the *sinus rhythm.* The SA node is the transformer of your heart house: It's where the electricity originates before it travels down the wires to the AV node, which acts like a junction box: It helps regulate the amount of electricity that can pass from the top chambers (atria or fillers) to the bottom chambers (ventricles or pumpers). This AV node or junction box, where the signal slows down, is the key regulator of electricity flowing to the ventricles. This important function of the AV node becomes even more important when there's an electrical problem in the heart.

One of the many amazing things about your heart's electrical system is that it's completely self-regulating. Assuming your heart is healthy and working well, it can sense the demands facing your body and adjust your heart rate accordingly—even to the extent of keeping up with your needs while you run a marathon, should you choose to do so. As your muscles draw on the oxygen and nutrients from your blood, your heart's electrical system ramps up to keep up with the increased demand, and your heart rate increases. The heart also detects when less is needed—for example when you're sleeping—and the rhythm slows accordingly.

A steady heart rate of 60 to 90 beats per minute is normal, though your heart's electrical system automatically increases this rate during physical activity and decreases it when you're sleeping. Six interconnected parts tell the heart when to contract, starting with the SA node, the heart's "natural pacemaker," moving to the upper chambers, then the ventricles, and back to the upper chambers where the cycle begins again.

CHAPTER 19

Rhythm Problems

Out of Rhythm

Michael took a walk in the park every day with his toy poodle, Maggie. He was in good physical condition despite being 79 years old. He lived on his own in a small apartment in New York City. He enjoyed strolling the neighborhood and taking in the lush greenery of the park every day. As Michael passed Joe and Charlie playing chess, he began to feel short of breath, which was unusual this early in his walk. His head started swimming, and he rested his hand on the corner of their table to steady himself because he feared he was going to faint. Charlie reached for Michael's forearm and gently helped him sit down. Worried that it might be something serious, the chess players called 911.

Michael's physical symptoms alone make it difficult to tell which particular heart complication he was experiencing. There's a fairly long list of things that can go wrong with your heart rhythm, some more common than others.

When your heart's natural ability to correctly pace itself begins to go awry, you have an "electrical system malfunction." The umbrella term for electrical problems is *arrhythmia*, which means an irregular heartbeat—one that's too fast, too slow, or erratic. Arrhythmias can be completely harmless and impossible to detect without specialized equipment, but they can also be immediately life-threatening.

If someone tells you they have an arrhythmia, tachycardia, bradycardia, skipped beats, palpitations, flutter, fibrillation, a pacemaker, or defibrillator, they're saying they have a problem with their heart's electrical system.

The severity of any heart rhythm issue is determined in part by its location. As you know, your Heart House is like a two-story building. If a non-load-bearing wall in a room on the top floor were to catch on fire, the damage would be relatively easy to manage. Emergency crews would put out the fire, you'd send in a repair crew, and the rest of the building would remain intact. On the other hand, if a load-bearing wall on the first floor were to catch fire, and if the structural integrity of the building were sufficiently compromised, the entire building could come crashing down. Remember that your heart's top chambers (the atria) work primarily as "fillers" in the cycle of your heartbeat, while the bottom chambers (the ventricles) are the "pumpers." Abnormal or inefficient pumping is more detrimental than abnormal or inefficient filling.

Electrical problems or arrhythmias come in two primary forms:

1. *Bradycardia:* too little electricity resulting in a heart rate that's too slow—fewer than 60 beats per minute
2. *Tachycardia:* too much electricity, leading to a heart rate that's too fast—more than 100 beats per minute

Electrical Conduction System of the Heart

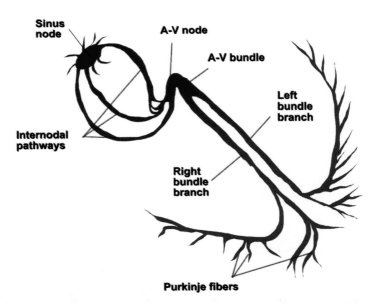

Bradycardias and tachycardias can result in symptoms such as palpitations, lightheadedness, or dizziness. Any one of the six parts of your heart's electrical system can operate at a rate that's too fast or too slow.

Bradycardia (Slow Heartbeat)

Imagine that you wake up one morning and the electrical system in your house isn't providing enough current. You yawn your way downstairs to brew some much-needed coffee, but when you flip the switch on your coffee maker, nothing happens. Your electrical system isn't keeping pace with the amount of electricity your home needs. This is, in essence, what is happening in your heart when you have bradycardia. Your heart requires full electrical power to do its job.

In general, it's better to have a slower resting heart rate because it's an indication of good cardiovascular health. But, if your resting heart rate is too slow, your heart may not pump enough blood to your brain, which can cause you to pass out.

> *Bradycardia is caused by a wire that's been damaged,*
> *and it causes a slowdown.*

There are several types of bradycardias, differentiated by the part of your heart's electrical system the problem where the problem originates:

- *Sinus bradycardia:* a problem with the sinus node.
- *AVN block:* a partial or complete interruption of the heart's electrical signal between the atria and the ventricles. There are three degrees of AVN block, ranging from first through third degree.
- *Left or right bundle branch block:* an interruption of the electrical signal somewhere in the right or left bundle branches.
- *IVCD (intraventricular conduction delay):* a slowing or block in the ventricular fibers.

Some individuals who are extremely physically fit (marathon runners, cross-country skiers, swimmers, and other endurance athletes) routinely have slower heart rates—below 60 beats per minute. It's also possible to have a slower than average heart rate even when you're not incredibly fit and still be perfectly fine. If you don't have any symptoms, that's likely the case.

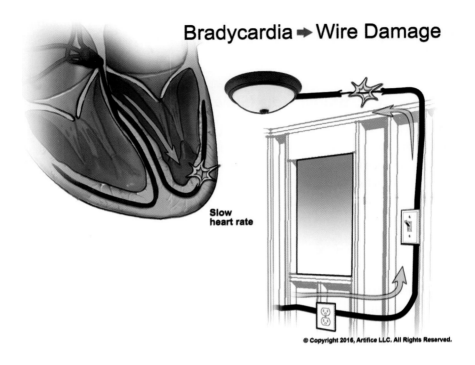

Bradycardia ➡ Wire Damage

Slow
heart rate

Tachycardia (Fast Heartbeat)

Worn or damaged wires can also prevent electrical signals from traveling smoothly, causing your heartbeat to speed up. The result is tachycardia: an abnormally fast heart rate of more than 100 beats per minute. As a consequence, the left and right ventricles may not have time to adequately fill with blood in between cycles. The symptoms of tachycardia can be similar to those of bradycardia: fatigue, dizziness, fainting, and shortness of breath. You may also experience a rapid pulse, a fluttering in your chest, chest pain, and heart palpitations (feeling like your heart is beating too hard or too fast). Think of tachycardia as a recurring electrical surge. When the electrical wires in your house receive an unexpected power flux, it can cause a relatively mild brownout or, in more severe instances, the surge can fry your outlets and appliances.

In some cases, an increased heart rate may not cause any problems other than slight discomfort when your heartbeat seems to flutter. Other times, tachycardia can lead to a stroke or could even be life-threatening.

Just as there are different types of bradycardias, there are numerous kinds of tachycardias. Each type's name reveals where it originates in the heart's electrical system. These abnormally fast heartbeats are broken down into two categories: *supraventricular tachycardia (SVT)* and *ventricular tachycardia (VT)*.

Supraventricular tachycardia is a fast heart rate that begins in the upper chambers of the heart:

- *Sinus tachycardia:* a problem with the sinus node.
- *AVN nodal tachycardia (AVNRT):* a problem with the AV node.
- *Atrial fibrillation* or *flutter:* a problem with the electrical fibers in the atria.

Ventricular tachycardia is a fast rhythm that starts in the heart's lower chambers (ventricles):

- *Left or right bundle branch ventricular tachycardia:* a problem or short circuit with the LBB or RBB.
- *Ventricular tachycardia:* a problem with the ventricles' electrical fibers.

Tachycardia is caused by a short circuit or worn insulation in the wires of your heart's electrical system, and it causes your heartbeat to speed up.

Syncope

We all know someone who's fainted. A sudden scare, extreme exertion, a quick drop in blood pressure because you stood up too fast, or even a violent coughing spell can be causes of "common faint," or *vasovagal syncope*. Most fainting is related to insufficient blood flow to the brain, which can occur when your blood pressure is too low, and your heart fails to pump enough blood to the brain to maintain consciousness. This leads to lightheadedness and fading vision, and progresses relatively quickly until the person loses consciousness.

Underlying this response is the vagus nerve, found at the base of your head; when this nerve senses that not enough blood is making its way to your brain, it prompts your blood pressure to drop. While fainting may seem like a counterproductive response, it acts as a natural failsafe in a simple if not graceful way: When you lose consciousness, you fall to the ground. Lying down allows blood to flow more easily back to your brain, which helps restore sufficient blood flow to the brain and restores consciousness.

Whether arrhythmias are slow or fast, they decrease the amount of blood that's pumped out of the heart, which in turns reduces blood flow to the brain and makes you pass out. Fainting related to heart rhythm disorders is called cardiac syncope.

There are other, less dangerous causes of syncope, including low blood sugar, but we have to run tests to determine why a patient passed out. If your primary care doctor refers you to a cardiologist because you've had a fainting spell, please don't think it's useless. You may have some form of cardiac syncope caused by an arrhythmia.

Fibrillation

Two specific electrical disorders, both called *fibrillations*, can be particularly serious because they cause the heart to beat erratically. *Ventricular fibrillation (VFib or VF)* is a common cause of sudden death or cardiac arrest, and *atrial fibrillation (AFib or AF)* is the most common cause of stroke in the elderly.

Ventricular Fibrillation (VFib)

Ventricular fibrillation is the most serious disturbance in your heart's rhythm and is life-threatening. VFib occurs in the lower rooms of your heart (the ventricles) when erratic electrical signals cause the ventricles to quiver. As a result, the heart can't pump blood, which causes cardiac arrest (sudden death).

Remember: There's a difference between cardiac arrest and a heart attack: A heart attack is a plumbing problem, while cardiac arrest is an electrical problem: Your heart stops beating, and you die.

Atrial Fibrillation (AFib)

Atrial fibrillation is a quivering or irregular heartbeat in the atria, the upper two rooms of your heart. One of the issues with AFib is that the ventricles tend to beat very fast in response to the erratic beating of the atria. AFib can lead to blood clots, stroke, heart failure, and other heart-related complications. At least 2.7 million Americans are living with AFib.[1]

Normally, the top chambers (atria) empty into the bottom chambers (ventricles), which pump the blood out to the body. In atrial fibrillation, this rhythm of events gets disrupted. The atria beat irregularly and can't move all the blood into the ventricles, so the blood stagnates in the atria. This stagnant blood has a tendency to clot. If a clot forms in the heart, it can be ejected out of the heart to the brain and cause a stroke.

Your heart naturally paces itself, but can have an "electrical system malfunction" (an arrhythmia). Damage to your heart's wires can result in a heartbeat that's too slow (bradycardia), too fast (tachycardia), or erratic (fibrillation).

CHAPTER 20

Causes of Rhythm Problems

Aging is the most common risk factor for electrical problems, but lifestyle choices and other underlying medical issues can also cause your electrical system to short out.

Aging

Just like the one in your house, the electrical system in your heart won't last forever, particularly if it's endured extra stress thanks to your lifestyle or genetic factors. But, even if you've made heart-healthy choices and aren't genetically predisposed to heart problems, your heart's electrical system may begin to show signs of wear, tear, and damage as you get older.

Similar events can take place in our heart's electrical system as we age. The older we get, the more likely we'll experience some degree of *fibrosis* or scarring. Depending upon the amount and depth of fibrosis, your electrical system might short out. In general, the greater the scarring, the less conduction your heart's electrical system will be able to sustain, and your power to keep blood moving throughout your body will weaken. Your doctor's job is to monitor this damage and prevent it from progressing to keep your electrical system up and running as it's supposed to run. Unfortunately, no one can avoid the effects of time, but we can be vigilant about getting regular checkups and addressing any problems before they get out-of-hand. That's why, if your doctor suspects any heart condition, an annual visit with your cardiologist is crucial.

Lifestyle Choices

By now, I'm sure you're not in the least surprised when I tell you that certain lifestyle behaviors can increase or decrease your chances of electrical problems. Obesity, excessive alcohol use, and the use of stimulants such as cocaine, caffeine, and cigarettes increase your risk for heart problems. You may have heard the term "Holiday Heart Syndrome," which refers to arrhythmias that occur in otherwise healthy people after they've imbibed too many drinks. Never underestimate the powerful effects our choices have on our bodies—and our future!

Other Medical Causes

Several medical conditions put you at a greater risk of developing arrhythmias: obstructive sleep apnea, obesity, and hypothyroidism, as well as heart issues such as coronary artery disease and heart valve disease. You're also at a higher risk for arrhythmia if you've had a heart attack. So, as you can see, taking good care of your heart house—and your overall health—significantly slashes your risk for arrhythmias.

CHAPTER 21

Diagnosing and Monitoring Rhythm Problems

New Mercedes

Let's face it: Some people don't trust their doctors any more than they trust their mechanic. You know how it goes: You take the car to the mechanic for a regular service appointment or to get something fixed, and they often add stuff to the invoice or suggest you have other work done, which doubles or triples the bill. And your response is, "Yeah, right!" Some people don't react much differently at the doctor's office.

Recently, I had a patient in my office who was preparing for knee surgery, which he desperately needed because he was struggling to walk even 10 steps without taking a break. Five years earlier his electro-cardiogram (EKG) had shown some abnormalities, so I thought it best to order an echocardiogram (echo) to make sure his heart could withstand surgery. Because this patient couldn't walk well, doing a standard treadmill stress test wasn't an option. Outside of the echo, I had no way of knowing if his heart was up to handling surgery. When I wrote the order for this test, my patient scoffed and said, "This is why I don't come to doctors. I guess you need a new Mercedes." Although it was easy for me to laugh it off, it's not easy to laugh off the risk my patient is taking with his health.

Many patients don't understand that even a non-cardiac surgery, say on the knee or hip, can increase their risk of having a heart event. More than 50 million surgical procedures are performed every year in the United States, and it's estimated that between 1.4% and 3.9% of them are complicated by a major cardiac event, such as a heart attack, stroke, or even heart-related death.[1] This risk can increase dramatically if you already have a heart condition, even if the surgery is performed nowhere near your heart.[2] So, it's not about a new car, but instead about controlling and understanding the risk before the surgery, rather than finding out after the fact that this elective knee surgery probably should have been postponed until after the patient's heart risk was addressed.

When a patient doesn't understand these things, they might take surgery lightly or think their physician is padding his wallet or being overly cautious. Admittedly, just as there are some mechanics who seize the opportunity to make a few extra bucks by performing unnecessary fixes on your car, there are doctors who go to sleep at night with visions of a shiny new Mercedes dancing in their heads. No one likes being ripped off, and the best way to safeguard against a shady diagnosis, whether at the mechanic's or the doctor's, is to become an educated consumer. Make sure those tests your doctor has ordered are necessary; make sure those fixes your mechanic recommends are needed. If in doubt—if you think that the motivation for either individual is their bank account—seek a second opinion. Money-hungry people exist in all professions; but believe it or not, most workers are truthful. I know many doctors, and I honestly think the majority are straightforward and want to do what's best for their patients. For the most part, doctors go into medicine for two reasons: first, to help people and, second, to challenge themselves in a demanding career. I think it's rare that someone opts to go into serious debt for eight years of schooling, another four to eight years of residency, fellowship, training, apprenticeship, and 16-hour workdays just because the pay is good.

If you have palpitations, lightheadedness, dizziness, or fainting, I start thinking of potential electrical problems. First I order the standard tests. The EKG measures your heart's electrical impulses. I order blood work to ensure you have a normal level of blood sugar and aren't anemic, and to be certain your thyroid and electrolytes (such as potassium and magnesium) are in the normal range. The echocardiogram is next so I can be sure that your heart is pumping enough blood to your body (especially to your brain), and that its walls and valves are healthy. If these standard tests don't show the reason for your symptoms, then it's time to move on to the focused testing for the electrical system.

You know how sometimes your car doesn't make the funny noise when you're at the mechanic? The same thing can happen with arrhythmias.

Monitors

Many arrhythmias happen only every so often, and may not show up on an EKG. To get more information about your heart's electrical function, we may ask you to wear a heart monitor (*Holter monitor*) for 24 or 48 hours.

Another option for monitoring heart rhythm is event monitors, which record your heart rhythm for seven to 30 days. They're similar to the Holter monitor, but have the capacity to hold up to 30 days of data. These can be helpful in diagnosing patients whose arrhythmia is intermittent or sporadic.

If your palpitations, dizziness or lightheadedness occurs only once a week, it's a waste of money to order a 24-hour Holter monitor because it likely won't show anything other than a normal rhythm. In this case, we use the 30-day event monitor, which gives us an opportunity to catch your sporadic symptoms. Sometimes, if patients have symptoms that make them pass out only once in two to three months, we use an *implantable loop recorder (ILR),* a device implanted under the skin of the chest near the heart. This little device records the heart's electrical activity on a continuous basis so that we can get minute-by-minute information on your heart's rhythm. The "electrician" doctor (electrophysiologist) implants the ILR. Using the ILR gives the doctor an edge: This device increases the probability that he'll catch abnormalities in your heart during episodes of dizziness or palpitations.

Mobile EKG

Another option is a *mobile EKG*. If you believe that modern day technology is still years away from developing some of the amazing gadgets you see in sci-fi films, think again. These amazing devices work using an app and a small pair of electrodes that you attach to the back of your smartphone. When you place your fingers on the electrodes, the device captures your heart's rhythm, and displays it on your phone's screen, providing immediate EKG data anywhere, anytime. Originally, this device was only available to physicians and other professionals, but now it's being sold directly to consumers. Of course, professional assistance is still needed to understand the results, so it wouldn't be a good idea to run out and buy one to diagnose yourself!

While your doctor may order more tests to see if the arrhythmia is related to other problems within your heart, the EKG is the most valuable tool for detecting the electrical activity of your heart.

The electrocardiograph, which measures electric current in the heart, has been around for more than a century: It was invented in 1903 by physiologist Willem Einthoven.[3]

The Electrophysiology Study

If all of the above standard diagnostic tools fail to uncover my patient's electrical problem, I then refer them to an electrophysiologist who can perform an *electrophysiology (EP) study.* This procedure is similar to the cardiac catheterization. However, instead of shooting dye in the arteries to detect a blockage, these catheters are designed to study the heart's electrical system. Using them, the electrophysiologist can determine if there's an arrhythmia in the heart, the cause, and extent of the problem—and even determine the best treatment. Depending on the results of the EP study, the electrophysiologist may continue with other procedures such as implanting a pacemaker.

Tilt-table Exam

Syncope is common in cardiac patients, but it presents a unique challenge to doctors because there are many cardiac and non-cardiac issues that can cause a patient to faint. When the results of all the standard tests (bloodwork, EKG, exercise stress test, Holter Monitor, echocardiogram, and EP study) are normal, only one test remains: the *tilt-table test.*

During the tilt-table test, the patient is securely strapped to a table while monitors for blood pressure and heart rate are placed on the chest. The technician or doctor then begins to tilt the table to a vertical position with the patient's head up. When the patient is tilted between 60 and 90 degrees, the doctor can tell if there's any association between the patient's body position and their symptoms. If the tilt test shows that the syncope isn't related to cardiac causes, we look elsewhere. Often, even after testing, we still don't know what could have caused the patient to faint. We call these cases *idiopathic*: it's a medical issue that has no apparent or known cause.

CHAPTER 22

Treating Rhythm Problems

Many of my patients with arrhythmias notice only mild symptoms now and then—nothing bothersome at all. I like to see these patients on a regular basis so I can keep an eye on things and make sure their symptoms aren't worsening or increasing in frequency; but for the most part, it's not worth the trouble of trying to correct the issue. When symptoms become more frequent or more debilitating, or if a patient's arrhythmia causes complications (like cardiac arrest or stroke), then we have to buckle down, find out exactly what's going on, and address it. The treatment for arrhythmias can differ depending upon whether the patient has bradycardia or tachycardia.

Bradycardias (Slow Heartbeat) Treatment

Doctors handle bradycardia based on causes and symptoms. When I discover a patient has bradycardia, I first look to rule out potential underlying causes such as hypothyroidism or medications like beta blockers or calcium channel blockers that can slow the heartbeat. However, the main reason people experience bradycardia is their age. Currently, no medications are available that reliably speed up a heartbeat that's too slow, so we insert a *pacemaker*.

Pacemakers

If you have a sluggish heart rate, particularly if you have frequent bradycardia that causes persistent dizziness, lightheadedness, or fainting, your doctor may suggest a *pacemaker*: a small device implanted in your chest that delivers electrical impulses to prompt the heart to beat 60 times per minute. Pacemakers are like backup generators. This invaluable mechanism can alleviate fainting and fatigue, and often allows the patient to resume a more active lifestyle. Pacemakers are implanted during a relatively straightforward procedure and generally hold up for the long term.

Tachycardia (Fast Heartbeat) Treatment

We have two goals when treating tachyrhythmia: reduce symptoms and reduce complications. We can do one of two things (or both) to reduce symptoms: control the heart rate or try to maintain normal heart rhythm. Treatment starts with medications and then if needed, we progress to using one of several procedures.

Let me give you an Artisan's Approach™ to treating tachycardias. Understanding each of these steps and discussing them with your cardiologist will help you craft a plan that works for you and takes into consideration the type of treatment you wish to have. (Every patient is different in this regard. For example, patients have told me they don't want a pacemaker: "If it's my time, then it's my time." I have to respect that. Each of us has our own belief system.) There are six modes of attack when trying to treat a fast heartbeat. Often doctors will use more than one approach depending on the effectiveness of the treatment or severity of the symptoms.

Step 1: Watch and Wait

It may sound crazy not to do anything, but if the short circuit comes once a year, you don't want to spend the money to have the electrician tape it up. When symptoms are rare, occurring only once or twice a year, I do nothing. I call it "watchful waiting." I may ask the patient to come back for checkups so I can keep an eye on things, and make sure the symptoms aren't getting worse or more frequent, but for the most part, treatment isn't worth the trouble.

Step 2: Rate Control Drugs

Sometimes, the "watch and wait" approach isn't the best fit for a patient, and a more proactive approach is required. Patients with frayed or damaged electrical wires may need rate control medications to slow the heart rate, reduce high blood pressure, and control arrhythmias. In that case, beta blockers such as atenolol and carvedilol, and *calcium channel blockers* such as diltiazem and verapamil are commonly prescribed. These medications decrease your heart rate by reducing the electrical impulses sent through the AV node. They belong to a class of medicines known as *AV blockers* or *AV-nodal blockers*. They help suppress the junction box or AV node, which in turn slows a patient's arrhythmias. They can suppress all six parts of the electrical system if needed.

An AV blocker is like the tape used to insulate frayed or damaged electrical wiring in your home. If an electrician sees only minor wear and tear on the outside of the wires, they don't rip out and replace all the wiring. Instead, they insulate the wires by wrapping them in electrical tape to ensure that the current continues to flow where it should. This saves you a lot of money and time. You doctor may instruct you to take these pills every day or sometimes just on the days you feel a rapid heartbeat. They're very effective when it comes to slowing down your heartbeat.

Step 3: Rhythm Control Drugs (Antiarrhythmic Drugs)

Unfortunately, some patients' arrhythmia can't be controlled with beta blockers or calcium channel blockers, so the next line of attack is to choose a stronger drug: an antiarrhythmic (AAD), which acts as the insulator. Examples of these drugs include flecainide (Tambocor®), propafenone (Rhythmol®), sotalol (Betapace®), and amiodarone (Pacerone®). These drugs are like heavy-duty insulation tape used to wrap high-voltage wires. In addition to providing more insulation, this group of drugs can help stabilize your heart's electrical system. These drugs help regulate and stabilize the voltage in the heart and prevent short circuits. It's crucial that patients who are on these antiarrhythmic drugs keep their electrolytes, potassium, magnesium, and calcium levels under close check with their cardiologist.

This class of drugs can make arrhythmias less frequent or severe, but these medications can also have side effects that make them difficult to tolerate.

Step 4: Cardioversion

Cardioversion is a procedure performed in the hospital that involves giving a brief, perfectly timed electrical shock to the heart through the chest wall. The goal is to disrupt the heart's abnormal electrical circuits and reset it to a normal rhythm. You won't feel any pain during this process and, since we give you some drugs to knock you out, you won't even remember it. During the procedure, your oxygen levels, blood pressure, and heart rhythm are closely monitored. It's an effective course of action, especially in emergency or life-threatening circumstances. But, since cardioversion isn't a cure—it's more like resetting the circuit breaker in your house— your arrhythmia can come back. So, even though your heart rhythm has been reset, doctors prefer to play it safe: After cardioversion, we usually prescribe antiarrhythmics or heart rate-lowering medications for most patients to help prevent recurrence.

Step 5: Implantable Cardioverter Defibrillator (ICD)

You may have a UPS (uninterruptible power supply) in your home. Often used to protect computers, a UPS is a device that allows a computer to keep running even when it's lost its power supply. An *implantable cardioverter defibrillator (ICD)* acts as a UPS for your heart. Unlike the kind of defibrillator that's used in emergency situations to jump-start your heart, the ICD is a small box that's surgically implanted beneath your skin with wires that run to the wiring of your heart, much like a pacemaker. It's used only to prevent life-threatening arrhythmias that occur in the lower part of your heart. When the ICD senses an extra surge, it sends out controlled impulses to help pace your heart. If that doesn't work, it delivers a larger shock of electricity, which restarts your heart. In a way, the ICD is similar to a generator wired into your house. If you've ever lived in an area with frequent power outages, you might have one. Once the power goes out, the generator kicks in, and life goes on—just as an ICD can ensure a person's life will continue when arrhythmias occur.

Step 6: Catheter Ablation

In the 1990s and 2000s, the defibrillator was the most common way to resolve a life-threatening fast heartbeat. Since then, technology and techniques have improved significantly. Now doctors have the option of removing the problem area through ablation. During an ablation procedure, an electrophysiologist, the type of cardiologist that specializes in arrhythmias, threads a small flexible tube through an artery in your leg or arm into your heart to destroy tissue that's creating the malfunction. The doctor can then stop the arrhythmia by burning out the area in which the rapid heartbeat originates.

Working inside the heart is a delicate process, and because there's a chance that the parts surrounding the problem area may become inadvertently damaged, cardiologists only want to go there as a last resort. There are plenty of risks involved if you think about it. The process is akin to cauterization, which uses burning to close a wound or remove damage—and burning an area of the heart is pretty extreme. It's comparable to hiring an electrician to work on wires inside the walls of your house. There's always the possibility that, because the wires are difficult to access, he may damage the drywall or plumbing surrounding the faulty wires. A good electrician will let you know whether or not this sort of work is necessary and will tell you what risks might be involved—and a good physician does the same.

It's important to work closely with your cardiologist to develop a treatment plan that you're comfortable with. I use my Artisan's Approach™ to collaborate closely with each patient to determine the best course of action, and I always keep in mind that what might be best for one might not be a suitable course of action for another. Working as a team ensures my patients maintain control, and I believe this approach leads to the highest rate of success.

VFib Treatment

Ventricular tachycardia, a fast, irregular rhythm, can lead to ventricular fibrillation, and must be treated. When ventricular tachycardia (VT) becomes too extreme to be treated by drugs, the next step is the ICD (implantable cardioverter defibrillator)—the same ICD we use to treat tachycardia.

When a person's heart is already in a life-threatening rhythm, an electric shock, administered via an external defibrillator, can restore the heart to its natural cadence. We've all seen countless examples of this on TV and in movies: the doctor puts the paddles onto the patient's body, yells "Clear!" and everybody steps back while the shock is delivered. Automated external defibrillators (AEDs) work the same way, but AEDs are designed to be used by people with little or no training and are made available in public places to help prevent deaths from cardiac arrest. AEDs automate the process somewhat: Once activated, they tell you exactly what to do, diagnose the arrhythmia, and select and deliver the proper amount of electrical current.

AFib Treatment

As with any arrhythmia that's not immediately life-threatening, cardiologists strive to reduce symptoms and complications when addressing AFib. Although the most dreaded complication of AFib is a stroke, we also work to prevent another complication: the weakening of the heart muscle caused by repeated or persistent arrhythmia. Over time, an erratic heartbeat takes a toll on overall heart function.

When it comes to treating AFib, I used a stepped, Artisan's Approach™, similar to my approach for dealing with tachycardia:

1. Watch and wait.
2. Rate or rhythm control medications.
3. Cardioversion.
4. Catheter ablation.

Step 1: Watch and Wait

In the early stages of AFib, I take a watch and wait approach, as episodes may be infrequent and may not bother the patient. However, AFib tends to be progressive, so episodes become more frequent over time. That's where my Artisan's Approach™ comes in.

Step 2: Rate Control Medications

Just as with any arrhythmia, when we treat AFib, we want to control your heart's rate and rhythm. The fast beating of the ventricles not only wears them, but also makes for an inefficient heartbeat because the ventricles don't have sufficient time in between beats to relax and fill completely. Slowing the heart rate with medication gives them time to relax and fill with blood. In addition to prescribing beta blockers and calcium channel blockers, we use *digoxin* to control AFib. Digoxin also slows heart rate, but it tends to work only when the heart is at rest so that you may need another medication in addition to it. These medications usually won't stop the AFib, but may reduce the symptoms of the arrhythmia to something more manageable or less noticeable.

Step 3: Cardioversion

If medication doesn't reset your heart's rhythm back to normal, then cardioversion is the next step. In addition to the same electrical cardioversion procedure we use in the treatment of tachycardia, we can perform a chemical cardioversion using an antiarrhythmic drug to convert the abnormal heart rhythm to a normal one.

Step 4: Catheter Ablation

The same *catheter ablation* that's used to treat tachycardia is used to treat AFib. An electrophysiologist threads a catheter up to the heart and burns certain areas, preventing electrical impulses that can trigger AFib. This procedure has been proven to reduce or eliminate the occurrence of AFib episodes. At first, researchers tested this procedure in patients who had more persistent or permanent AFib than the "average" AFib sufferer. But, doctors discovered that catheter ablation seemed to work well—better than other techniques or available drug therapies—so they extended its use to "less sick" patients. Now, people who have milder forms of AFib benefit from this procedure. Doctors hope that treating patients earlier will prevent some of the chronic long-term damage caused by arrhythmia.

Thanks to this innovation, many former AFib sufferers are free from arrhythmias or have significantly fewer or shorter recurrences. Very few who've undergone catheter ablation have experienced complications, though some patients have had to undergo the procedure a second or third time to treat their AFib fully. With the advent of catheter ablation, we hope to see a reduction in pacemaker implants and medication.

Pacemaker

The pacemaker is an exception to my stepped Artisan's Approach™ when it comes to AFib. Sometimes the drugs used to slow your heart work too well, and your heartbeat might slow down too much. In this case, you may also need a pacemaker to keep your heart at a sustainable rate. Once you have a pacemaker, your doctor will adjust your medications to best manage your symptoms. A pacemaker is also used for *tachy-brady syndrome,* a condition in which the heart sometimes beats too slowly and other times too quickly. This type of arrhythmia is often seen in patients with AFib.

Blood Thinners

To prevent the blood from clotting and causing a stroke in AFib patients, we prescribe blood thinners. Once again, my Artisan's Approach™ comes in. Aspirin is the most commonly used blood thinner and many patients who are diagnosed with AFib already take aspirin to prevent stroke and heart attack. I determine whether you're safe on aspirin alone or need a stronger blood thinner based on your particular circumstances. Just because your cousin has atrial fibrillation and her cardiologist has prescribed aspirin, while your cardiologist has prescribed warfarin for you doesn't mean the two doctors' recommendations are contradictory. You may have additional risk factors for stroke such as diabetes, congestive heart failure, or coronary artery disease.

Depending on each patient's circumstances, I may prescribe the anticoagulant drug warfarin (Coumadin®) for AFib patients, or one of a class of newer drugs called *NOACs* (novel oral anticoagulants). NOACs, such as dabigatran (Pradaxa®), rivaroxaban (Xarelto®), and apixaban (Eliquis®), are associated with less bleeding than some of the older medications, so many cardiologists are abandoning the old drugs and prescribing these new ones for their AFib patients. Most patients can take anticoagulants for years, even decades, without experiencing any issues. However, depending on the particular medications you've been prescribed, you may need to be regularly monitored at your doctor's office to make sure your blood isn't being thinned too much. For example, Coumadin® requires close monitoring, but NOACs do not.

Problems with the heart's rhythm can be treated with medications, devices such as pacemakers, and surgical procedures—or, in some cases, not treated at all. The right treatment for you depends on the type of arrhythmia you have and the severity of your symptoms.

CHAPTER 23

Rhythm Lifestyle Tips

Many lifestyle habits can cause your overall heart health to deteriorate, but certain behaviors are especially risky for your electrical system. Smoking is dangerous to your health, whether we're talking about your heart's plumbing system, its electrical system, or any other part of your heart or body. It's just an unhealthy, nasty habit, and if you smoke, you need to quit. While smoking won't necessarily cause an arrhythmia, it will certainly make it worse by unnaturally increasing adrenaline. Quitting smoking is always a good health decision. Period.

Speaking of unhealthy substances, some substances can impact your heart's electrical system, even when used in moderation. These include alcohol, (a depressant that can act as a stimulant), and other stimulants, which can throw off your electrical system, especially if you've had arrhythmias in the past. I've already mentioned the dangers of overuse of alcohol, but recent studies have suggested that even moderate drinking can increase atrial fibrillation, the most common form of arrhythmias.[1]

Stimulants that can cause cardiac arrhythmias include cocaine, amphetamines, methamphetamine, ephedrine, cold medicine, and even some medications for ADHD. One study of children who were taking Ritalin and similar drugs indicated that they were at a 61% higher risk for arrhythmias in the first two months of treatment compared to children not taking these medications.[2] Illegal drugs such as cocaine and over-the-counter cold medicines can predispose patients to unpredictable tachycardia as well as bradycardias.[3] Caffeine is the most common stimulant linked to arrhythmias.

If you're on antiarrhythmic drugs, see your cardiologist every six to 12 months for close monitoring. The same goes if you have a history of heart disease or arrhythmia and are taking prescribed stimulants. And, avoid over-the-counter or recreational stimulants altogether: if you have any form of tachyarrhythmia, cut out alcohol and caffeine. Any amount of alcohol or caffeine can provoke a tachycardia attack.

1. Quit smoking: It's your body, so make good choices even if you have to ask for help.
2. Cut out excess alcohol and caffeine: Moderation is the key.
3. Avoid any illegal stimulants and recreational drugs: That's not a road you want to travel.
4. Consult with your doctor if you're taking prescribed drugs: Stay on top of your heart health.

PART 6

The Valves: Your Heart's Doors

CHAPTER 24

How Your Valves Work

The doors in your house allow people and things to pass from room to room, as well as in and out of the house itself. The *valves* in your heart function in a similar fashion: Just like the doors to your bedrooms and bathrooms, they open and close. They allow blood to flow from one chamber of the heart to the next, and then close tightly to prevent backflow.

Your heart valves are composed of strong, thin flaps of tissue called leaflets or cusps. For the valves to work properly, they need to be properly formed and fitted together. They also need to open and close fully.

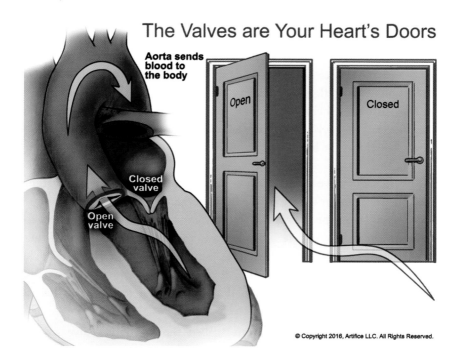

The Valves are Your Heart's Doors

The doors in your heart operate in a slightly different manner from the doors in your home, however. While the doors in your house usually open in only one direction, they allow traffic to flow both ways. When all is working as it should, your heart valves also open in only one direction, but they're more restrictive: blood can flow only one way. Think about entrance and exit gates at an amusement park. If people ignore the signs and go against the flow of traffic, what happens? You end up with a huge traffic jam, no one able to move in or out as people work against each other. Heart valves prevent this from happening, which is good: Our blood needs to circulate for us to survive.

Your blood follows a crucial route that carries oxygenated blood to every part of your body. Remember that your heart is like a two-story duplex with two rooms on each floor. The two rooms on the top floor are the atria; they receive blood flowing back to the heart. The two rooms on the bottom, the ventricles, pump blood out of the heart. The doors (valves) control the flow of blood through the heart by opening and closing as the heart contracts.

A normal heart valve is about the size of a half dollar. The beating sound of your heart is the clap of the valve leaflets opening and closing.[1]

There are four valves in the heart, connecting atria to ventricles and regulating the blood flowing out of the heart. Each must open completely to allow the right amount of blood to flow through at the right time, and then close tightly to prevent blood from flowing backward. These four valves (in the order that blood flows through them) are the *tricuspid valve*, the *pulmonary valve*, the *mitral valve*, and the *aortic valve*. Let's take a look at how these valves regulate the flow of blood in the heart and through the body:

- The tricuspid valve is the door between the right atrium (the upper right room) to the right ventricle (the bottom right room). It opens to allow the blood that's just flowed into the right atrium (from the body) to pass to the right ventricle. Then it closes to prevent blood from flowing back into the right atrium when it's pumped out of the right ventricle to the lungs. As the name implies, the tricuspid valve normally has three leaflets, but it's not the only valve that's formed this way: The aortic and pulmonary valves also generally have three flaps.
- The pulmonary valve, sometimes called the pulmonic valve, is the passageway between the right ventricle and the pulmonary artery—in

other words, it's the exit door to the lungs. When it's closed, it allows blood to enter the right ventricle from the right atrium without any escaping prematurely to the lungs; when it's open, it enables blood to flow to the lungs to obtain oxygen.

- The mitral valve is the doorway from the left atrium (the upper left room) to the left ventricle (the lower right room). It's the only valve that's composed of two leaflets, so it opens like a French door. After blood has picked up oxygen in the lungs, it returns to the heart, flowing into the left atrium. The mitral valve opens to allow blood to flow from the left atrium into the left ventricle, and closes to prevent blood from flowing back into the left atrium from the ventricle.

- The aortic valve is the door out of the left ventricle. It opens and closes to regulate the flow of oxygen-rich blood from the ventricle out through the aorta and to the whole body. Although the aortic valve usually has three leaflets, in 1 to 2% of the population it has only two leaflets (*bicuspid aortic valve disease*).[2] In those who have this disease, the valve doesn't work optimally, but may work well enough that it doesn't cause noticeable symptoms for many years.

CHAPTER 25

Valve Problems and Symptoms

When the doors in your house don't open and close properly, people and things can't pass through as they should. For example, in the summer, when the doors stick, it's a struggle to pull them open when you need to walk from room to room or close them completely when you want privacy. In the winter, when the door and the frame contract due to the cold, air can flow through the cracks, creating drafts in the house. Imagine if the valves in your heart began functioning this way. If they didn't close or open properly, they might allow blood to leak, or prevent blood from flowing through unrestricted. Leaky and poorly functioning valves (doors) are types of *valvular heart disease.*

The most common symptoms of a poorly functioning valve are also the most common symptoms of problems with the heart's plumbing and walls: shortness of breath, lightheadedness, dizziness, passing out, fatigue, and even chest pains. You may feel short of breath because blood is entering your lungs the wrong way, or experience chest pain because parts of your heart aren't getting the right amount of blood. You may also notice swelling in your hands and feet because your blood is going backward all the way to your extremities, causing them to retain fluid. As is the case with other heart-related problems, the symptoms may not always indicate which part of the heart is malfunctioning. Your cardiologist needs to do a battery of tests to tease out the real cause.

Sometimes a valve fails slowly, allowing the heart to compensate bit by bit to the subpar performance of one of its parts. In these cases, a patient might not recognize that they have symptoms of valve disease because they have gradually limited their daily activity levels over a period of time.

People want to think that their heart is like that famous bunny that just keeps going and going, but potential heart problems shouldn't be ignored. Any of your heart valves can become damaged and work poorly, though you should be particularly concerned if the *aortic* or *mitral* valves malfunction. These two valves perform critical tasks by controlling the circulation of blood to the farthest extremities of your body. They work under higher amounts of pressure than the valves on the right side of the heart, which are only involved in regulating the blood flow to the lungs. The aortic valve, for example, helps control the flow of oxygenated blood out of the heart. Obviously, a problem with this valve could be catastrophic. Damage to the *tricuspid* and *pulmonary* valves carries less severe consequences than a similar amount of damage to the aortic and mitral valves.

Heart Murmurs

***If your doctor tells you he hears a heart murmur, don't panic!
There's a chance it's nothing to be concerned about.***

Many people panic when they're told they have a *heart murmur*, but it's not always a cause for alarm. A heart murmur is simply an extra or unusual sound heard during a heartbeat, and can be caused by stuck or leaky doors. Even if your valves are perfectly normal and healthy, they might make an audible sound if you push more blood through them than usual, or push it through faster than normal. The sound—often a whooshing or whistling—is caused by blood moving through an opening creating turbulence. While heart murmurs are often related to valve problems, not all murmurs are problematic or need to be treated. When a heart murmur is considered non-threatening, we call it an *innocent heart murmur*. For instance, during pregnancy, a woman gains 10 to 15 pounds of blood. As this extra blood tries to move efficiently through the body, the valves make more noise than they normally might. A fever may also cause an innocent heart murmur. Also, young children can get heart murmurs while going through a growth spurt. Even exercise can create a temporary heart murmur, as it increases the speed at which blood flows through the heart.

Sometimes, though, this sound is a sign of trouble. Heart murmurs that are cause for concern include those that result from congenital heart valve defects and acquired heart valve disease, such as valve stenosis and regurgitation.

Valve Regurgitation

Regurgitation is backward flow through a valve that isn't closing completely. If a heart valve is damaged or ill-fitting, a small amount of blood slips back through the valve in the wrong direction when the heart pumps blood out of the chamber. When the aortic valve doesn't close properly, some of the blood that was just pumped out of your left ventricle leaks back into it. This is known as aortic valve regurgitation. Similarly, mitral valve regurgitation occurs when the mitral valve doesn't close properly, allowing blood to leak back through it into the left atrium.

Regurgitation can be dangerous because it can allow deoxygenated blood to flow to your body and oxygenated blood to return to your lungs. If the problem is severe enough, it can cause *cyanosis*, a condition in which the skin, lips, and fingernails develop a bluish tint because the blood flowing from the heart to the body isn't carrying enough oxygen.

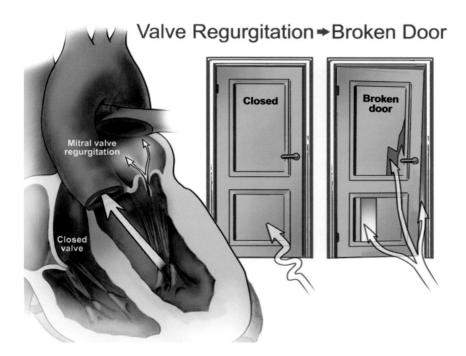

Valve Stenosis

Stenosis is a constriction or narrowing that prevents the valve from fully opening, like a stuck door in your house. A *stenotic valve* is like that door that's jammed: It can't open fully to allow blood to flow freely. Because the valve isn't allowing enough blood to flow through it, the heart has to work harder to pump the same amount of blood. Eventually, this increased workload takes an even more serious toll: After years of pumping harder, the heart begins to weaken (*valve-induced cardiomyopathy*), which in turn causes valve-induced heart failure.

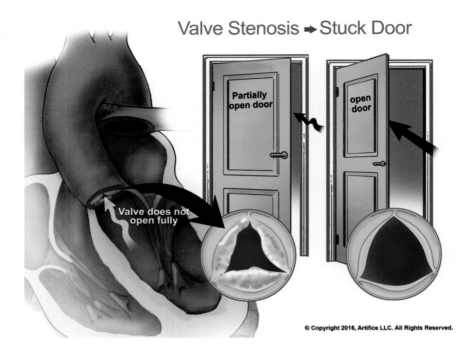

Valve Stenosis ➡ Stuck Door

Partially open door

open door

Valve does not open fully

© Copyright 2016, Artifice LLC. All Rights Reserved.

Aortic stenosis is the most common heart valve disease related to calcification, and it's the one I see most often in my patients. The aortic valve operates under more pressure than any other valve, and when calcium begins to build up on the flaps of this valve, it has a more pronounced effect than damage to the valves on the right side of the heart. A stenotic aortic valve may reduce the volume of oxygenated blood that reaches the rest of the body. Initially, the left ventricle thickens as it tries to keep up with the extra load, a condition known as *left ventricular hypertrophy*. Eventually, a stenotic aortic valve may reduce the volume of oxygenated blood that reaches the rest of the body.

In mitral valve stenosis, the flow of blood to the left ventricle, (the main pumping chamber), is blocked because the valve doesn't open as wide as it should. Some people can feel fine with valve stenosis, while others experience symptoms such as shortness of breath, feeling tired, and heart palpitations. Symptoms will typically get worse with an increased heart rate. The main cause of mitral valve stenosis is rheumatic fever.

Malfunctioning valves can be jammed or leaking. Jammed valves don't open fully (stenosis), while leaking valves let the blood go the wrong way (backflow or regurgitation). The aortic valve works the hardest of all the valves, so it's at the highest risk of becoming damaged. If it does become damaged, it carries the most life-threatening outcomes. The usual suspects of chest pain, shortness of breath, and fatigue accompany valve issues, but your doctor may also hear a heart murmur.

CHAPTER 26

Causes of Valve Problems

Now that we understand what a heart valve is, and what can potentially go wrong with it, the next logical question is: *Where do these problems come from?* The answer often depends on your general health history, your age, and which valve is causing you problems.

The most common causes of valvular heart disease are age-related calcium buildup in the valves and congenital conditions. In many people, the heart valve tissue naturally deteriorates with age until the valve can't function properly. So, even if your valves once worked just fine, as you get older, the tissue may begin to break down and calcify. High blood pressure and atherosclerosis (a disease in which plaque builds up in your arteries) may hasten this process, but that's not the case with everyone. And as with several other heart conditions, some people are born with congenital valve abnormalities that cause problems right away or later in life.

Calcification

As a house ages, you can expect to have to repair or replace some of its original features thanks to normal wear and tear and the aging process. The same happens with your body as you age. No matter how health-conscious you are, certain changes occur. Calcification is a natural and mostly unavoidable process in which calcium salts begin to accumulate in the body's tissues, causing them to harden. This can happen anywhere in your body, including in the arteries of the heart, and in your muscles, breast tissue, bones, or teeth. Kidney stones and gallstones are often caused by calcium deposits. Calcification is a normal part of aging, and the most common cause of valve defects that I see in my patients.

Rheumatic Fever

Untreated strep infections can progress to rheumatic fever and can cause *rheumatic heart disease*: inflammation and scarring in the heart. This condition is triggered by an autoimmune reaction to the infection and can show up during the acute phase of the infection as inflammation of hearts walls (myocardium) or doors (valves). When valves become inflamed they may become damaged or scarred, though this scarring and damage often remain undiagnosed for many years until the individual develops stenosis or regurgitation later in life.

Not so long ago, rheumatic fever was the most common cause of acquired heart valve damage, though today this disease is almost unheard of in most developed countries, thanks to the widespread availability and use of antibiotics. It's still a significant cause of valvular heart disease in some places, however.

Congenital Defects

Congenital defects can cause a leaky valve with either regurgitation or stenosis. Earlier in life, these abnormalities may not cause any signs or symptoms other than a heart murmur, but as a person ages, these issues can become more serious or urgent.

One of the most common congenital valve conditions is pulmonary valve stenosis. Sometimes the only sign of this type of stenosis is a heart murmur; when this condition is mild or isn't causing symptoms, it doesn't need to be treated. However, severe pulmonary valve stenosis needs to be addressed as it can require the heart to work harder, leading to heart failure. In another form of congenital valve defect, the three leaflets that form the valve are malformed or fused, creating two leaflets instead of three. This is the case in bicuspid aortic valve disease. As a result, the valve isn't as sturdy as it would otherwise be and can't function as well as it should.

Bacterial Endocarditis

Beyond aging and rheumatic fever, there are several other causes of acquired valvular heart disease. One is *bacterial endocarditis*, an infection of either the inner lining of the heart (the endocardium) or the heart valves. Endocarditis occurs when viruses or bacteria from another part of your body, such as your mouth, enter your bloodstream and settle on damaged areas of the heart. Bacteria circulating in your bloodstream don't stick to the inside of a healthy heart; but, if your heart valves are abnormal, or your heart tissue is damaged in some way, the bacteria can attach to these areas. Bacterial endocarditis is uncommon, but can be life-threatening if left untreated.

Before the medical world discovered the many applications of penicillin, cardiologists commonly recommended complete tooth extraction for all patients at risk of infection-related endocarditis and valve disease. Unfortunately for these poor patients, most cases were caused by specific bacteria, and could have been cured by penicillin. Think about how many teeth could have been saved![1]

Other Causes of Valvular Heart Disease

Usually, I see heart disease in one area of the heart at a time. For example, blocked plumbing causes chest pain. Cardiomyopathy is a problem with the heart walls. However, sometimes problems in one area of the heart can cause problems in another area: For example, problems in your heart's walls and plumbing can lead to problems with the valves because these systems are connected, just as they are in your house. If your plumbing is blocked, your pipes may burst, which can lead to damp walls that eventually warp. Warped walls no longer provide a good fit for the doors, and the doors can't close tightly.

Fen-phen is one of the substances that can be detrimental to your heart's valves. In the 1970s, a pharmaceutical company released a diet pill containing fenfluramine, but it wasn't very popular or widely used because it only helped reduce weight temporarily. In the 1990s, however, this company combined fenfluramine with phentermine, creating the drug we commonly refer to as "fen-phen." The company began heavily marketing the product, citing efficient, drastic, and long-lasting weight loss. Unfortunately, this particular combination of drugs has the adverse effect of attacking the heart's valves in a way similar to the effect of rheumatic fever. As fen-phen enters your bloodstream and passes through your valves, it corrodes and attacks them, making them unable to close properly.

You may be wondering about the legal diet pills that have flooded the market over the last couple of decades. While regulating bodies like the FDA have given the companies that manufacture these drugs their stamp of approval, in truth, few studies have revealed what they do to your body over an extended period. I know many of you don't want to hear this, but it's best to avoid diet pills altogether. No magical and safe cure-all drug exists. If you want to lose weight, do it the old-fashioned way: Focus on diet, exercise, and other lifestyle changes. Luckily, when you get heart healthy, you're making changes that help you lose weight and become whole-body healthy as well.

 Valve disorders can be caused by aging, rheumatic fever, genetic defects, certain infections, calcium, and old diet meds. Natural is always best. When trying to lose weight or up your calcium, try going with whole foods. When that isn't sufficient, you owe it to your overall health—not just your heart health—to work closely with your doctor instead of experimenting on your own.

CHAPTER 27

Diagnosing Valve Problems

As I mentioned earlier, patients with valvular heart disease may have a heart murmur, feel unusually tired or short of breath, or notice swelling in their ankles, feet, legs, or abdomen. But, some have no symptoms at all, and the problem is only discovered when they have a chest X-ray or other imaging test to check for an unrelated issue. Cardiologists often make decisions regarding treatment based on both the patient's symptoms and the results of imaging tests, which can reveal how serious a valve problem is. Some patients don't notice any symptoms at all, and in these cases, reliable imaging tests help physicians determine the best course of action.

As with all heart conditions, we first order the standard tests: an EKG, bloodwork, and chest X-rays. The specific tests we use to learn more about a patient's heart valves involve the use of *ultrasound*, a safe and painless procedure that uses high-frequency sound waves (echoes) to produce pictures of the heart. (Ultrasound is also called *sonography.*)

Echocardiography

An echocardiogram (often called an "echo," not to be confused with an EKG or *electro*cardiogram) is the most common test used to confirm that a patient has valvular heart disease. An echo looks at the heart's structure using ultrasound waves, which pass through a device (a transducer) placed on your chest. The echo from the sound waves (as they pass through your chest wall) is converted by the machine into pictures of your heart. This test can show whether your heart valves appear normal in shape and size, how well they're working, and if there's backflow through the valve.

Doppler Ultrasound

Doppler ultrasound (sometimes called Doppler echocardiography) is similar to an echo. It's the test of choice when your cardiologist hears a heart murmur because pictures produced by the sound waves show blood flow, and alert your doctor to any leakage of the heart valves.

Imagine you're in a railroad station, waiting to board. While you're standing there, you hear a train passing by. You can tell by the sound when the train's coming toward you and when it's moving away because the intensity of the sound waves changes. Using this principle, doctors can tell how serious a murmur is, based on the sound of blood going through the open valve.

Transesophageal echocardiography

Before cardiologists put patients through a major heart surgery, we like to have a close look at the appearance and function of the heart. *Transesophageal echocardiography* (TEE) is a way to look closely at the valves. Like a traditional echo, TEE uses sound waves, but the transducer is attached to the end of a flexible tube, which is guided down your throat and into the esophagus. From this position right behind the heart, we can get a much better view of your heart and its arteries. It's not the most comfortable procedure, but it's tolerable: You'll be given medication to both numb your throat and help calm jittery nerves before the test. There's little risk to this examination beyond the possibility of having a sore throat for a few days afterward. Some cardiologists' offices and hospitals use a 3-D technology that enables us to view real-time 3-D pictures, and study the heart in greater depth than we've ever been able to before. I use 3-D technology whenever I perform an echo or a TEE.

Most general cardiologists are trained to perform both TEE and echocardiography. TEE is a big part of echocardiography, and requires its own board certification. Doctors have to be highly trained and specially licensed to pass the board examination and get the okay to practice TEE. (Remember I said that I tell my patients I'm a part-time photographer? I'm referring to my role of taking pictures of the heart. I'm certified in both echo and TEE and was thrilled to introduce TEE to my hospital's cardiac unit.)

Good doctors spend a lot of time and effort studying for certification tests so they can perform these types of diagnostic examinations. It's not easy to achieve multiple certifications and it's always a good idea to know which ones your doctor has.

CHAPTER 28

Treating Valve Problems

Unfortunately, much like wall damage, malfunctioning valves can't be cured with a quick fix. But, not all valve issues require surgery.

Non-Surgical Options

In the section on your heart's walls (Part 4), we talked about the four types of drugs that help reduce symptoms and, in some cases, reverse mild damage. However, there is no drug that can dissolve scars (from rheumatic fever, for example) or regrow damaged valves. Dermatologists and cancer researchers have found drugs that can be injected into scars to decrease their burden in other areas of the body. However, we can't use them on the heart because it's moving and beating; these drugs might cause a short circuit in the wiring of the heart, which could cause the heart to abruptly stop beating (known as *cardiac arrest*).

Some valve damage is mild enough that the patient can live with the minor symptoms. In these cases, doctors monitor the patient and do regular echocardiograms to keep an eye on how the damage is progressing. In moderate to severe cases, doctors may also suggest that this individual limit strenuous activities such as weightlifting and running.

Some valve issues (like mitral stenosis) can raise the risk of blood clots; for them, we prescribe anticoagulants ("blood thinners") to prevent clots. As is the case with any cardiovascular issue, a heart-healthy lifestyle is recommended to patients with valvular heart disease. Although avoiding situations and activities that stress the heart in general or raise blood pressure is always important, it's especially vital when the heart is already damaged. And, yes, I know it's not always possible given the complex world in which we live.

Surgical Options

When the symptoms of a valve problem become more severe, or the issue becomes more life-threatening, a surgeon needs to step in. Unlike heart walls that will slowly heal over time once the cause is removed, the valves, once damaged, will remain damaged forever. Surgery is usually required for severe stenosis of the aortic and mitral valves. If the cardiologist feels valve replacement surgery is needed, they may order a cardiac catheterization test to confirm that this operation is necessary. (Catheterization involves sending a small tube through the veins to assess the state of the heart's arteries and valves.) By the way, during the cardiac catheterization, the cardiologist can assess the heart's plumbing as well. Plumbing and valve problems can be taken care of during the same surgery.

Valve replacement and repair surgery accounts for 10 to 20% of all cardiac procedures.[1] However, even though this type of surgery is fairly routine, I'm not claiming it's without risk. After all, we're talking open-heart surgery. Earlier I mentioned that aortic stenosis was the most common heart valve disorder I see in my practice. Two-thirds of all heart valve operations are performed to remedy this condition.[2]

Repairing Valves

Heart valve repair is recommended if the surgeon feels the valve can be repaired, and that it will last a long time. For example, the mitral valve can often be repaired as opposed to being replaced. Surgeons take several approaches to valve repair surgery. They may be able to repair the existing heart valve by adding tissue to increase the support at the base of the valve or to patch holes or tears. Or, they may reshape the valve by stitching it so that it closes more tightly. Sometimes, if the flaps are fused together, a surgeon can separate them so that they can move freely and work more effectively.

Replacing Valves

If you need a valve replacement instead of repair as is often the case with the aortic valve, the surgeon has to decide whether to use a *bioprosthesis* or a mechanical prosthesis. Of course, there are pros and cons to both. Bioprostheses come from pig, cow, or human heart tissue. These valves don't tend to last as long as mechanical prostheses, but they've been specially treated so that you won't need to take blood thinners (anticoagulation drugs) for the rest of your life to prevent your body from rejecting the valve. On the other hand, mechanical prostheses are durable, but require a more extensive regimen of monitoring and medication—including blood thinners—to prevent the body from rejecting them.

> ***If you hear someone say they have a pig or bovine valve,***
> ***they're talking about an issue with one of the doors of their heart.***

Recovery from valve replacement surgery may be a long process. However, most patients find that their symptoms subside quickly. During and after recovery, it's important that patients follow the recovery and lifestyle plan recommended by their cardiologists to avoid future issues.

Transcatheter Aortic Valve Replacement (TAVR)

In the last several years, a less invasive means of replacing a damaged valve has been developed and tested, and it's now rapidly being adopted worldwide. *Transcatheter aortic valve replacement* (*TAVR*) involves using a catheter that's threaded through an artery (often the femoral artery in the groin area) and extended up to the heart. Currently, this minimally invasive surgery is the only valve treatment that can be done on a beating heart. At the tip of the catheter is a deflated balloon with a folded replacement valve connected to it. Using the catheter, a surgeon can place the valve in the proper position and then expand the balloon to secure the new valve within the old valve. The balloon is then deflated and removed, along with the catheter. Because TAVR is much less invasive than traditional valve surgery, it has opened the possibility of valve replacement to many more patients, including those considered too weak or sick to undergo a full-fledged surgical valve procedure.

The transcatheter valve technique is most developed for the aortic valve. But interventional cardiologists (plumbers), those who specialize in these less invasive, catheter-based (or *trans*catheter) techniques, are working on ways to treat other valves (namely, the mitral valve and the pulmonary valve) with similarly less invasive procedures.

As with all new procedures (and most older procedures too, for that matter), TAVR doesn't have a perfect track record: Some patients have experienced leakage and backflow around the valve. Though TAVR isn't for everyone, I feel it's worth exploring with my patients if they need an aortic valve replacement. Once again, I put my Artisan's Approach™ to good use as, together, the patient and I examine all options available and make an informed decision based on his or her unique situation.

CHAPTER 29

Valves Lifestyle Tips

Valve problems are not the result of lifestyle, and there are few, if any, lifestyle changes you can make to improve the health risks to your heart's valves. Age, rheumatic fever, and congenital defects are beyond our control—unless you've somehow miraculously discovered the Fountain of Youth. (In which case, I'd like to become your best friend.) Seriously, the most you can do is be vigilant about your health and maintain safeguards, especially when you deal with other health professionals. They need to know your complete medical history, no matter how minor you believe those conditions are.

However, few people think that going to the dentist is a big deal, but dentists, like other medical professionals, need to know exactly where you stand health-wise—including the medications you're taking—and be familiar your medical history before they deal with your dental problems. Dentists aren't worried that you're going to have a heart attack during a simple cleaning, but they are concerned about heart murmurs and infections. During certain procedures like tooth extractions or root canals, your dentist often digs, drills, and scrapes teeth and gums that are coated with decades of plaque and may be heavily infected. The major concern is that the bacteria causing your tooth infection could enter the blood stream and head straight to your heart. If it does, and you have an existing heart murmur, the bacteria is more likely to get stuck in your heart and cause bacterial endocarditis. If you warn your dentist of your condition, he can prescribe antibiotics before surgery. This preventive measure can go a long way in mitigating the infection before it becomes an issue.

Not everyone agrees with the preventive use of antibiotics, but the American Heart Association has promoted the practice and even encouraged individuals to carry a "preventive infection" wallet card that can be filled out by your doctor. (You can find the wallet card on the American Heart Association website at www.heart.org.) I've always been an advocate for preventive health measures, and I guarantee that if you carry the card, you and your dentist will thank me! Plus it will save you an extra trip to the cardiologist and prevent any delays in your dental surgery. Who knows? That card might even save your life.

1. Take illness seriously. If you have a known diagnosis and get a fever, this could be the beginning of life-threatening infective endocarditis.[1]
2. Tell your dentist. If you have a history of a heart murmur or endocarditis, don't keep it a secret.
3. Carry the preventive infection wallet card. If you have a murmur, this card lets your other health care providers into the loop so they can decide whether or not to prescribe antibiotics as a safety measure.
4. Stay on top of rheumatic fever. If you or a loved one had rheumatic fever as a child, make sure your doctors know so they can monitor the heart valves closely.

PART 7

The Pericardium: Your Heart's Siding

CHAPTER 30

How the Pericardium Works

Just as your house has siding that insulates it and protects the exterior walls, your heart does, too: it's surrounded by a fibrous membrane that serves similar purposes. The siding of your Heart House is known as the *pericardium*.

It serves four purposes:

1. Keeping your heart in place.
2. Preventing your heart from expanding too much when its blood volume increases.

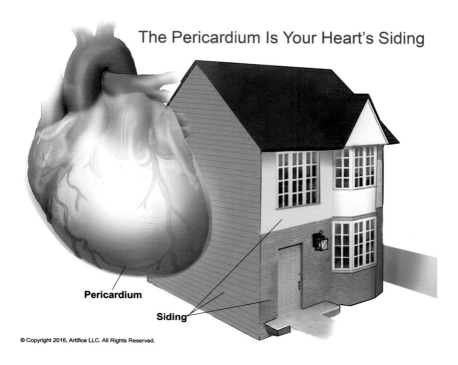

The Pericardium Is Your Heart's Siding

Pericardium

Siding

3. Lubricating the heart while it expands and contracts during the pumping cycle.

4. Preventing infections in other organs, such as the lungs, from spreading to the heart.

The pericardium has two layers. The outer layer, the *parietal pericardium*, anchors the heart in place: it attaches to both your diaphragm and breastbone. This outer layer of siding also connects to your lungs, so it holds your heart and lungs close to one another. The inner layer, the *visceral pericardium* or *epicardium*, is two layers in one, with one layer closely surrounding the heart itself and the other attached to the outer layer. The space between these two inner layers is called the *pericardial sac* and is filled with fluid that acts as a cushion for the heart.

CHAPTER 31

Problems with the Pericardium

Most of the time an issue in your heart's siding isn't nearly as life-threatening as an issue with the plumbing, walls, or electrical system, though some pericardial conditions can be extremely dangerous. As is the case with problems in many other areas of your heart, chest pain is typically the first symptom of issues in the pericardium. Since your pericardium is so close to your lungs, this pain can feel worse when you cough or take a deep breath. Depending on your particular type of pericardium woes, you may also experience fever, trouble breathing, fatigue, and weakness. In general, the symptoms of siding issues can also be signs of other types of heart problems, and the only way to be sure of what's causing them is to see your doctor.

When your heart's siding has problems, it's like your house's siding having problems: It may be bad, but it's not as bad as a problem inside the house would be.

Compared to other parts of the heart, the pericardium is subject to relatively few problems. *Pericarditis* and *pericardial effusion* are the most common issues by far.

Pericarditis
Not a Heart Attack

Mike made his way through the aisles of the grocery store, grabbing boxes of cereal and graham crackers for his 5- and 7-year-old daughters. As he reached for the milk, he felt a sudden wave of dizziness. He brushed it off as a fluke, but as the shopping trip drew to a close, he found himself growing more and more tired for no apparent reason, and he struggled to push the cart through the checkout line. When he made it home, he apologized to his wife and lay down. While he was resting, he began to have trouble breathing, and felt a sharp pain start in his chest and shoot down his left arm. The pain worsened as he struggled to take deep breaths and became increasingly short winded. "This is it," he groaned. "This is the big one. I'm having a heart attack." In a panic, he told his wife to call 911. A short time later, an emergency room physician quickly determined Mike wasn't having a heart attack after all, but the doctor needed to conduct more tests to pinpoint exactly what was happening. Mike underwent several diagnostic procedures, including bloodwork, chest X-rays, electrocardiograms (EKGs), echocardiograms, and ultrasounds, and the doctor concluded he had pericarditis.

As the name implies (with *–itis* at the end), pericarditis is inflammation of the pericardium. Mike's pain was caused by the layers of his pericardium rubbing against his heart. A doctor can hear this "pericardial rub" using a stethoscope. Chest pain and pressure are the most common symptoms, though pericarditis can also cause nausea, low-grade fever, fatigue, and trouble breathing. The pain of pericarditis gets worse with movement, deep breaths, or coughing because the movement of the lungs irritates the pericardium where it's attached to the lungs. Patients often feel better when they bend forward as this helps separate the inflamed layers of the pericardium.

Let's say you go to your doctor complaining of chest pain. Of course, as all good doctors would do, he'd listen to your heart and ask you specific questions about the nature of the pain. For instance, he'd want to know whether the pain is more a jabbing sensation or a dull throbbing feeling, if it's worse at certain times, and so on. Using this information, your physician may be able to tentatively rule out an angina attack or acid reflux, and zero in on the probable cause—pericarditis. For example, if you're in more pain when you move or take a deep breath (we call this "pleuritic" pain), there's a good chance that pericarditis is the cause.

Pericarditis can last for as long as several months and its onset is usually acute, which means this particular affliction develops suddenly. The condition also is somewhat rare: only about 5% of all people who arrive at the emergency room with non-heart attack related chest pain are diagnosed with pericarditis.[1]

The most common cause of pericarditis is a viral infection that makes its way to the heart, causing inflammation in the siding. Other causes include autoimmune diseases, injury to the chest, or a recent heart attack or heart surgery. However, most of the time pericarditis is considered *idiopathic*. While I like to joke that this means that the doctor is an idiot and the patient is pathetic, it's just a fancy way of saying we don't know the cause. Many cases of idiopathic pericarditis are presumed to be triggered by viruses, but it's not always cost-effective to run tests to determine which one has brought on the infection—especially because knowing the cause of the infection doesn't change the treatment.

Unfortunately, pericarditis often becomes a recurrent disease, which means if you've had one attack, you may have another down the line. Up to 30% of people who suffer acute idiopathic pericarditis will have a relapse at some point.[2] Chronic pericarditis (which begins gradually and lasts for a long time) is less common, but it's harder to deal with because it can persist for years despite treatment.

Perhaps you live in an area of the country that experiences a lot of rainy, damp weather. After some years in your house, you notice that the siding is buckling in spots, and begin to smell a faint musty aroma. Furthermore, a disgusting green mold is creeping up the siding on the shady side of your house. You call a repair man who assesses the damage and says, "If you don't fix things now, they'll only get worse. You don't want these conditions to spread to other areas of the house. I can contain the current damage and repair the siding now, but you'll always have to keep an eye out for future mold, mildew, and buckling issues because you live in a wet climate. You need to pay close attention and keep on top of problems as they arise."

Likewise, if you receive a diagnosis of pericarditis, you and your medical team will need to keep an eye on your heart health if your illness reoccurs.

A kitchen faucet would have to be turned on all the way for at least 45 years to equal the amount of blood pumped by the heart in an average lifetime. And, the heart is capable of squirting blood at a distance of up to 30 feet.[3]

Pericardial Effusion and Tamponade

A healthy pericardium contains a few tablespoons of fluid between its layers, but sometimes an infection, chest injury, or autoimmune disease will result in an excess buildup of fluid. This excess fluid buildup is called *pericardial effusion*. Though infection is a frequent cause of pericardial effusion, people who've had heart attacks or heart surgery may also experience this problem. The abnormal amount of fluid puts pressure on the heart. Since the heart's siding doesn't stretch very easily, if the fluid builds up too quickly and places additional pressure on the heart, this vital organ may be unable to fill completely with blood. This condition is known as pericardial or cardiac *tamponade.*

Pericardial effusions are relatively common. While pericarditis is the most common cause, many diseases and conditions may also be the culprit. Effusions are common after cardiac surgery, though they usually resolve on their own within a few weeks or months. Since pericarditis and effusion go hand in hand, the symptoms of effusion are the same as those of pericarditis: fever, fatigue, muscle aches, chest pain, and shortness of breath.

In each of these pericardial conditions, your immune system reacts with inflammation to stave off infection and damage. Once this inflammation sets in, the pericardium can become thick, and if the area between the heart wall and the pericardium becomes inflamed, the heart wall can suffer damage. An even more severe complication known as *chronic constrictive pericarditis* can set in if the inflammation becomes ongoing, causing scarring and damage to the heart muscle.

CHAPTER 32

Diagnosis and Treatment of Pericardial Problems

Treating problems of your heart's siding often focuses on preventing the issue from getting worse. But if fluid is already building up in your pericardium, your doctor may need to take a more aggressive approach.

Pericarditis

If I suspect you have pericarditis, I usually listen for a pericardial rub with a stethoscope and order an EKG. These simple diagnostic tools will reveal if you have any abnormal heart rhythms that typically occur during pericarditis, as well as help me rule out a heart attack. Other tests I might use to confirm that you're experiencing pericarditis include:

- blood tests (which can evaluate if there has been damage to the heart itself).
- a chest X-ray (which shows if your heart is enlarged or your lungs are congested).
- an echocardiogram (which shows how the heart is functioning and can point to pericardial effusion).
- a cardiac computed tomography (CT) scan (which detects any fluid or inflammation).

Sometimes I also order a cardiac catheterization, which measures the pressure in your heart as it fills, to see if the pericarditis has constricted the heart's ability to pump. This procedure is performed mainly for chronic pericarditis patients.

Treatment for pericarditis focuses on reducing inflammation and preventing effusion or tamponade. Once I have a sure diagnosis of pericarditis, I typically take a layered approach to treatment, depending on how severe the inflammation is when you're evaluated.

If the inflammation is in its early stages and not causing other complications, I prescribe an *NSAID* (nonsteroidal anti-inflammatory drug) such as ibuprofen or aspirin. Recent studies have shown that *colchicine* (an anti-inflammatory originally used to prevent pericarditis from returning) may also be an effective treatment for acute pericarditis, and that using it in combination with an NSAID is more effective than using either drug alone and reduces the chance of recurrence.

Pericardial Effusion and Tamponade

If I think a patient has pericardial effusion, then by now, you know what's next: tests! After examining the patient, the standard tests to check for pericardial effusion include an echocardiogram, electrocardiogram (EKG), and chest X-ray. The echo allows me to see the amount of space between the two layers of the pericardium, which tells me the extent of the pericardial effusion. If it shows decreased heart function, then I know the patient also has tamponade. The patterns of the EKG can also suggest tamponade. And finally, if there's a significant amount of fluid in the pericardium, a chest X-ray will show an enlarged heart.

First and foremost, the treatment of pericardial effusion is focused on preventing this condition from progressing to the point that it prevents the heart from filling or pumping. If fluid is building up in the pericardial sac, a patient may need to undergo *pericardiocentesis*, an ultrasound-guided procedure that drains the excess fluid from the pericardial sac using a large needle. General cardiologists, interventional cardiologists, and heart surgeons are trained in this procedure, and some emergency room and intensive care unit physicians may also be qualified to carry out a pericardiocentesis. It's an intricate procedure that's only performed on patients who already have tamponade or are at significant risk for developing it, and great care is taken to avoid puncturing a lung. Once the fluid's been drained, the symptoms begin to subside, and there's little lasting damage.

If the fluid buildup persists after pericardiocentesis, physicians need to take a more aggressive surgical approach to draining the fluid. This entails a procedure called a *pericardial window*, a surgical incision that makes a hole through which we can drain the fluid. If the window created by the surgeon is under so much pressure that it's unable to drain, we might need to perform an even more aggressive procedure: open the chest and cut out a piece of the pericardium. This is called *pericardial stripping.* Once the pericardium has been removed, the danger and pain are relieved.

It may take a few weeks or even months to recover fully from pericarditis or pericardial effusion. With close monitoring and rigorous treatment, however, patients often recover with few lingering effects.

While the siding of your house isn't the most important structural or functional piece of your house, it serves an important purpose. Similarly, the siding of your heart doesn't receive nearly the attention that the plumbing, electrical, or even the walls do, but it acts as an added buffer from infection and keeps the heart in place.

CHAPTER 33

Pericardium Lifestyle Tips

Since the biggest danger to your heart's siding can be caused by a viral infection, preventing an infection is the key to keeping your pericardium healthy. In addition to fastidious personal hygiene, all of the immunity-boosting habits that ward off the flu or the common cold also work to help you avoid pericarditis.

Stress can play a huge role in your heart health. When you're worried or overwhelmed, *catecholamines* (hormones your adrenal glands make in response to stress) are released into your blood stream. Your body immediately reacts by increasing your heart rate, constricting your blood vessels, and tightening your muscles.[1] While this response can be beneficial during competitions or in threatening situations, our bodies weren't designed to maintain high levels of these hormones for sustained stretches of time. A constant influx of adrenaline and norepinephrine cause high blood pressure, an increase in cholesterol, and an overall decline in heart health.

How do we manage stress so it doesn't have costly side effects? The first answer is meditation. Regular meditation has profound effects on your mindset, self-esteem, outlook, and mental stability. As your mental well-being becomes more in tune, your body also finds balance. The mental and physical health benefits of meditation are numerous and well-documented. Most importantly for your heart health, meditation has been shown to reduce stress and improve high blood pressure. Often, patients get started by focusing on their breathing or use guided relaxation techniques.

The second way to manage stress is to get enough sleep. It seems like such common sense, but one in three adults don't get sufficient shut-eye.[2] Inadequate sleep has been shown to lead to higher blood pressure, clogged plumbing, heart failure, heart attacks, stroke, diabetes, and obesity.[3] To compound matters, lack of sleep increases stress—which in turn puts you at even greater risk for a host of heart issues.

Getting enough sleep, on the other hand, reduces stress. Establishing healthy sleep routines can help you get the rest you need. Try to go to sleep at the same time every night, and turn off your electronics at least 30 minutes before you plan to head to bed. Keep your bedroom dark and cool. Once your bedtime has become a habit, getting enough sleep will be a welcome relief.

1. Let go of stress—it isn't serving any healthy purpose.
2. Start a meditation practice to find balance in your life through mindful awareness.
3. Get some sleep! Turn off the electronics, create a routine and go to bed.

PART 8

The Aorta:
Your Heart's Driveway

CHAPTER 34

How Your Aorta Works

I like to call the aorta the "driveway out of your heart." It's the largest artery in your body, (about a foot long and just over an inch in diameter), and through it, oxygenated blood leaves your heart and moves to the rest of your body. The aorta begins at the top of the left ventricle, which you may recall is the bottom left room of your Heart House. Since there's only one road out of the heart, you can imagine how important the health of the aorta is to your overall well-being and conversely, how dangerous it is if this artery tears or springs a leak. *All* of the arteries, including those that feed the heart itself, branch off from the aorta.

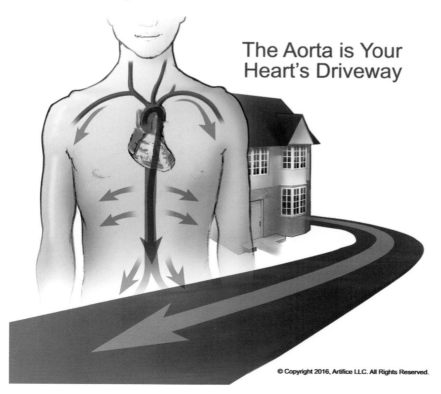

The Aorta is Your
Heart's Driveway

The aorta itself is divided into two main sections: the *thoracic aorta* is located above your diaphragm, which sits just above your stomach and below your ribs. (When I refer to the aorta being a driveway, I'm referring primarily to the thoracic aorta.) The *abdominal aorta* is the section from the diaphragm down. As a cardiologist, I diagnose, study, and treat problems of the thoracic aorta.

I jokingly tell my patients that my medicine stops at the belly button. Even though I was trained in vascular medicine, the field of medicine that looks at the body's arteries and veins, I refer patients with aorta problems to my vascular surgeon colleagues, who are the experts on the driveway. Unlike the cardiothoracic surgeon (the carpenter in our Heart House analogy), the vascular surgeon is a specialist, more like a concrete mason who specializes in fixing the driveway.

The thoracic aorta is further divided into three segments:

- As its name suggests, the *ascending aorta* reaches upward from your heart and is about two inches long. The right and left coronary arteries (the coronary artery system, which supplies blood to the heart itself) branch off this part of the aorta.

- Above the ascending aorta is a curved section known as the *aortic arch,* which is shaped like an upside-down "U." The right and left common carotid arteries, which carry blood to your brain, are branches from the aortic arch. The right and left subclavian arteries—those that take blood to your arms—also stem from the aortic arch.

- Past the arch is the *descending aorta*, which (not surprisingly) reaches downward through the chest. This part of the aorta hugs the back. Once it reaches the diaphragm, its name changes to the abdominal aorta. All of the arteries that send blood to your body from the chest down branch off of the descending and abdominal aorta.

Your aorta serves as the driveway out of your heart. It's your body's main artery and supplies blood to your entire circulatory system.

CHAPTER 35

Aorta Problems and Symptoms

You'd think that your driveway would represent a relatively safe place, sort of a quiet haven before the beginning of a journey—an area where you can let down your guard because you're still within mere steps of your house. But unexpected catastrophes can happen in driveways just as they can on any pathway. Two very serious problems can arise in the aortic driveway out of your heart: aneurysms and dissections. Both can rupture and be life-threatening.

Aortic Aneurysms

Your blood speeds through the highways of your body like cars on the freeway. It travels to the heart so it can be sent to the lungs to pick up oxygen, then back to the heart again, where it's pumped out of the well-traveled driveway of your Heart House.

 The heart pumps oxygenated blood through the aorta (the largest artery) at about 1 mile (1.6 km) per hour. By the time blood reaches the capillaries, it is moving at around 43 inches (109 cm) per hour.[1]

Unlike the driveway of your house, which can only accommodate a specific number of vehicles at one time, your aorta can stretch to make room for extra traffic. This is perfectly normal. But—just as the passage of time, excessive use, and other factors can cause wear and tear to your driveway—sometimes the walls of your aorta weaken due to aging, atherosclerosis, or *cystic medial necrosis,* a disease involving cyst-like spaces in the muscle fibers of the aorta. When your aorta's walls grow weaker, they lose their ability to stretch and can no longer withstand the pressure of an increased volume of blood. So, rather than expanding, the aortic wall begins to bulge outward, forming an *aneurysm.* An aneurysm can develop anywhere in the aorta so that you can have a *thoracic aortic aneurysm or (TAA)* or an *abdominal aortic aneurysm or (AAA).*

Symptoms of Aortic Aneurysms

Both types of aneurysms can grow so slowly that many people exhibit no symptoms. When symptoms do occur, however, that's usually a strong indication that the aneurysm is growing at a rapid rate. Some patients can actually feel a growing aneurysm putting pressure on nearby organs. For instance, if a thoracic aneurysm (in your chest) swells enough, it can compress the nearby lungs, making you feel short of breath; it can also irritate the nerves supplying your vocal cords, making your voice hoarse. You might also experience heaviness or pressure in the chest. A fast growing abdominal aortic aneurysm may also display certain symptoms: As the aneurysm increases in size, it may press on the nerves in your back, causing a feeling of discomfort and pressure. You may also suffer constant pain or fullness in your abdomen. Sometimes, pulsations from very large aneurysms can be felt near your belly button. It's rare, but if you're thin enough, you or your doctor may be able to feel these pulsations simply by putting a hand on your stomach. However, if you're obese, this warning sign may be missed. Perhaps that little tidbit of knowledge will provide an incentive for some readers to lose weight!

The scary thing about aneurysms is that they can pose a grave danger to your heart health—or even your life—because they don't always remain harmless bulges. Sometimes, if an aneurysm grows large enough, it will rupture—a condition that's immediately life-threatening. Each beat of your heart pushes a significant amount of blood into your aorta, and if your aorta has a hole, much of that blood leaks out rather than traveling to where it's needed throughout your body. Unless a ruptured aneurysm is stopped almost immediately, it will likely lead to shock and then to death from internal bleeding.

Aortic Dissection

You drive in and out of your driveway day after day and year after year, barely noticing the small crack that's appeared—until, one day, that small crack isn't so small. Instead, a huge piece of pavement has separated from the driveway, and rivulets of rainwater pour into the widening crevasse. If you don't repair this immediately, you'll end up with a completely washed out driveway and a river where the pavement once stood. This is hazardous.

An *aortic dissection* occurs when a tear forms in the innermost layer of the aortic wall. Blood leaks into the aortic wall through this tear, causing the layers of the wall to separate, and blood can flow in between the layers of the aortic wall, creating a dissection. The pressure of the blood flow often causes the dissection to expand, further disrupting the layers of the aortic wall and compressing the area through which blood can travel normally. As the blood continues to collect within the wall of the aorta, the wall can become weak and bulge outward or rupture if it's not treated quickly. An aortic dissection is one of the most dangerous conditions that cardiologists detect and treat.

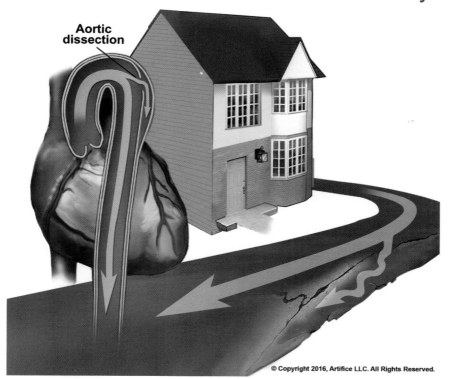

Aortic Dissection ➡ Cracked Driveway

There are two main types of aortic dissections. Cardiologists use the Stanford classification, which designates an aortic dissection as either "A" or "B." The Stanford type A aortic dissection affects the ascending aorta and arch; it's a medical emergency. Since the arteries that carry blood to the heart and brain branch off of these upper parts of the aorta, problems in these areas can prevent your heart and brain from getting the blood they need to function. The Stanford type B dissection occurs in the lower part of the thoracic aorta and isn't nearly as dangerous. Here's my easy Artisan's Approach™ to remembering the difference between the two types of dissections: Type A refers to a dissection involving the **a**scending **a**orta and/or the **a**ortic **a**rch, both of which begin with "A"; Type B involves the descending aorta, which runs down the **b**ack, which begins with "B."

Symptoms of Aortic Dissections

Unlike aneurysms which don't always have symptoms—unless they grow to a large size—aortic dissections usually cause severe pain, often described as a "ripping" or "tearing" feeling. It usually begins in the chest and radiates to the upper back, between the shoulder blades, or sometimes down the arms or to the neck. Some patients describe this as "crushing chest pain," making it difficult to distinguish from the pain of angina or a heart attack. Other non-specific symptoms, all the result of limited blood supply, include anxiety, dizziness, clammy or pale skin, nausea, and rapid or weak pulse, making it hard to diagnose a dissection by just taking a history and observing symptoms.

> *If you feel severe crushing chest pain radiating to your back, neck, shoulder, or jaw, immediately call 911.*

The location of your pain can reveal what type of dissection you have. The most common symptom of type A dissection is sharp, knife-like chest pain that sometimes radiates to your back. Type B dissections involve the part of the aorta that hugs the back, and cause pain that originates in your back and radiates to your chest. So, sudden, sharp pain in your back or in between your shoulder blades could be a sign of a dissection in your descending aorta.

 There are two problems that can occur in the aorta: an aneurysm or a dissection. Both can rupture and be life-threatening. Aneurysms remain silent unless they grow big enough for doctors to detect during an exam, or for patients to experience symptoms. Dissections are classified into two types: Stanford A and B. Stanford type A is a medical emergency.

CHAPTER 36

Causes of Aorta Problems

I doubt you'll be surprised to learn that circumstances and actions that increase problems in one area of your Heart House can do the same in other areas. As a matter of fact, in addition to wreaking havoc with your plumbing, atherosclerosis or plaque can lay waste to your driveway by triggering aortic aneurysms and dissections. Plaque builds up in your aorta for the same reasons it forms in the arteries of your heart. Aging, poor diet, smoking, high blood pressure, high cholesterol, and not enough exercise can all lead to an increase in plaque in your aorta. High blood pressure is the number one cause of aortic problems not only because it increases your risk for plaque, but because it causes your blood to push outward on the aorta. If the pressure of the blood that comes out of your heart is too high, it puts stress on the walls of the aorta.

The same lifestyle factors that affect your plumbing also affect your aorta because it's the biggest artery that comes out of your heart.

Individuals with certain inherited connective tissue disorders, such as *Marfan syndrome,* or bicuspid aortic valve defects are more likely to have trouble with their aorta. Abdominal aortic aneurysms (AAA), more common than thoracic aortic aneurysms (TAA), are usually caused by atherosclerosis, though they can also be caused by infections.[1] Thoracic aortic aneurysms are typically caused by high blood pressure or sudden injury.[2]

CHAPTER 37

Diagnosing Aorta Problems

Aneurysms remain silent until they grow large. Then they scream. The U.S. Preventive Services Task Force recommends one-time screening for abdominal aortic aneurysm (AAA) with ultrasonography if you are between the ages of 65-75 years and have ever smoked.[1] There's no routine screening for thoracic aortic aneurysms (TAA) unless you have symptoms or a family history of TAA.

Diagnosing problems in the aorta begins with the standard tests, including an EKG, bloodwork, and chest X-ray.

Aortic Aneurysm

Cardiologists use echocardiograms, transesophageal echocardiography (TEE), CT scans and MRIs to screen for and monitor aortic aneurysms. Of course, we don't order all these tests at the same time. We opt for echocardiograms and TEE, two types of ultrasound, if we want to avoid contrast (dye) and radiation. But, if we can't make a diagnosis based on those two tests, and there are no concerns about using contrast (dye) for a particular patient, we resort to both a CT scan and an MRI, which allow us to spot a bulge in the aorta.

Screening for Thoracic Aortic Aneurysms

Since conditions that cause a thoracic aortic aneurysm sometimes run in families, your doctor may recommend that you be screened for thoracic aortic conditions even if you don't have any symptoms. For example, you may be given tests if a first-degree relative (such as a parent, sibling, or child) has *Marfan syndrome*, a connective tissue disease. These tests may include imaging tests and possibly genetic testing.

Many famous people have suffered from Marfan syndrome including Julius Caesar and Abraham Lincoln.[2]

Aortic Dissection

If a patient arrives at the ER and the doctor suspects an aortic dissection, a contrast chest scan is ordered immediately. This is the gold standard. However, if a patient can't tolerate the contrast dye used in this test due to kidney disease or an allergy, we can also use transesophageal echocardiography (TEE) to view the heart. If a type A dissection is confirmed, the patient goes into surgery immediately for repair of the dissection.

CHAPTER 38

Treating Aorta Problems

The larger the diameter of an aneurysm, the more likely it is to rupture. So the way we treat an aneurysm depends on how big it is, as well as on a patient's other risk factors. Dissections are treated with emergency surgery.

Aortic Aneurysm

Once your cardiologist determines that you have an aortic aneurysm, he must decide if the aneurysm should be immediately repaired or if a "wait and see" approach might offer a better alternative. Obviously, a small aneurysm (less than 5.5 cm) doesn't pose the same risk of rupturing as a larger one, so he could decide to monitor the aneurysm's growth on a regular basis and prescribe beta blockers to help decrease the speed of growth.

In addition to medication, your doctor will suggest changes in your lifestyle that are crucial if you wish to prevent or inhibit the growth of aortic aneurysms: Quit smoking, or don't start. We know smoking is linked to the rapid expansion of aneurysms, as well as their rupture. I also prescribe other lifestyle changes such as exercise, following a healthy diet, and limiting alcohol. Sometimes we prescribe medicine for high blood pressure and high cholesterol to keep the risk of a heart attack or stroke at bay.

If your aneurysm is larger, between 5.5 cm – 6.0 cm, your doctor may suggest you undergo a procedure to repair it. An Artisan's Approach™ is used here as well: Every case is unique, and there is no "one size fits all" solution. The doctor must weigh the benefits and risks of a repair for each individual. People are living, breathing beings—not robots. They can't be "fixed" like a manufactured part on an assembly line. I look at the potential dangers of the procedure and consider how likely an aneurysm is to rupture, and balance that with the patient's overall health and ability to withstand surgery. I also consider a patient's gender and lifestyle, as these factors can make a patient more likely to experience a rupture. Women face a higher risk than men, and smokers are also more prone to rupture.

If your abdominal aortic aneurysm must be repaired, your doctor will speak with you to determine the type of surgery you need: traditional, open surgery or a newer, minimally-invasive procedure called *endovascular aneurysm repair option* (*EVAR*). EVAR involves making incisions in the groin area, and using catheters and dye to view your aorta on an X-ray during the procedure. A man-made tube called a stent graft is used to repair the aneurysm.

If your aneurysm has ruptured, you must be treated immediately. Even during and after repair of a rupture, the risk of death is high.

Aortic Dissection

Since type A aortic dissections can prevent blood from flowing to your heart and brain, they're treated with emergency surgery—the same EVAR procedure that's used to repair an aneurysm.

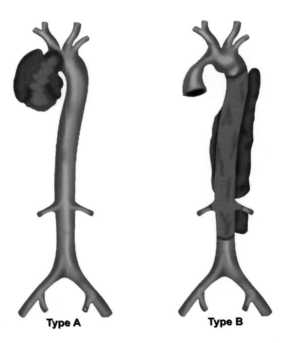

Type A   Type B

Type B dissections are typically treated with medicines, and by managing risk factors, especially high blood pressure as this condition increases the pressure on the aortic wall, making the tear more likely to grow. Doctors often prescribe beta blockers to patients with dissections that aren't at high risk for rupture. And of course, we routinely monitor patients with type B dissections. Surgery for type B is rare; but such a procedure may be called for if the aorta has ruptured, if the pain can't be controlled with medication, or if there's damage to other organs.[1]

CHAPTER 39

Aorta Lifestyle Tips

Your aorta is an artery—the largest in your body—so it stands to reason that the same lifestyle changes that benefit your heart's plumbing also help keep your aorta healthy. Hypertension is the biggest risk factor for both aneurysms and dissections, so keeping your blood pressure low is the surest way to prevent dangerous aortic complications.

Diet is a big factor in keeping your blood pressure in check. In previous chapters, I touched upon the importance of eating more fruits and vegetables and less red meat, sodium, and sugar. Luckily, there's a diet that caters to these exact recommendations: the DASH (Dietary Approaches to Stop Hypertension) diet. Though it was developed by cardiologists specifically to help heart patients reduce their blood pressure, those who followed this diet ended up losing weight, increasing their good cholesterol and stabilizing their heart health. The DASH diet (www.DashDiet.org) provides guidelines and sample menus for incorporating more fruits and vegetables, learning portion control and reducing salt.

The DASH diet also helps patients eat a healthy amount of fiber. Fiber doesn't just help your digestion: it's also vital to your heart as it lowers your blood pressure, removes bad cholesterol, and helps you reach or maintain a healthy weight. By increasing your intake, you can lower your risk of a stroke by up to 36% and your risk of type 2 diabetes by up to 30%.[1] Fiber is found naturally in whole foods like the fruits and vegetables I love talking about so much, as well as in whole grains, beans, and nuts. Adults should get between 21 and 38 grams a day (depending on age and gender) to reap the benefits.[2]

1. Maintain a healthy blood pressure: Get your blood pressure checked regularly and ask your doctor for advice on lowering it if it's high.
2. Start the DASH diet, the perfect eating plan for heart health.
3. Practice portion control. Even if you're choosing healthy foods, eating too much will lead to unhealthy weight gain.
4. Get enough fiber. Eat plenty of whole, plant-based foods.

My Aspirations for You

So … together, we've reached the end of this book. I trust your journey through its pages was educational, and you've learned a lot about your Heart House, its six parts, their critical roles, and how they all function together to keep you ticking!

I don't pretend the book is exhaustive, but I believe that it provides readers a solid platform from which to develop a deeper understanding of the heart. Armed with this knowledge, you'll be better equipped to understand your diagnosis or that of a loved one, and participate in making decisions about treatment. There's so much information on the Internet—some of it is incorrect and misleading—and some of it is reliable. Having read this book, you're now better prepared to determine the difference.

If you're ever diagnosed with heart disease, I hope you'll feel more comfortable being an active participant—and not just a bystander—with your cardiologist, when it comes to making decisions about your treatment. Together, you and your doctor can take an Artisan's Approach™.

I also hope this book will be a reminder to my fellow clinicians and me that, like the forefathers of medicine envisioned, medicine should remain a science *and* an art—the art of healing people. Each of us is built differently. Just like your house is different from mine, your Heart House is unique! An assembly line approach to caring for your heart doesn't result in the care that's best for *you.*

> *It takes more than science, nurses, doctors, and even self-help*
> *books such as this one to heal a person. It takes an approach*
> *that views each patient as unique and treats them as*
> *individuals—an Artisan's Approach* ™.

My heart will sing if I learn that—with the knowledge gained in *Your Heart House*—just one reader has been able to take an active, informed role in the care of their heart. It's my desire that readers will be able to assist doctors in walking that fine line of balance between science and art. This approach—an Artisan's Approach™—results in an individualized treatment plan for you or your loved one, with the best scientific basis as a backbone.

Please join me in my journey to discover new problems, create solutions, educate the masses and preserve mankind.

This is what we Hindus call "Aadi," the beginning of something important.

Connect with the Author

I urge my readers to ask questions, join the discussion, and find more information on my website and blog:

YourHeartHouse.com

I want to hear from you!

Acknowledgments

Writing a book is not a solo undertaking. I would like to express my sincere thanks to my family, and the many people who accompanied me on the journey of turning this book from a dream into a reality. I'm grateful to all those who provided support, talked things over, read, wrote, provided feedback, and assisted in the editing, proofreading, and design.

And to Nupur ... I could never have done it without you.

References

A Note to My Readers

1. Heart Disease and Stroke Statistics – At-a-Glance. American Heart Association website. http://www.heart.org/idc/groups/ahamah-public/@wcm/@sop/@smd/documents/downloadable/ucm_470704.pdf. Updated December 17, 2014. Accessed August 25, 2016.

2. Heart Disease Statistics. American College of Cardiology website. https://www.cardiosmart.org/Heart-Basics/CVD-Stats. Accessed August 31, 2016.

Chapter 3: Causes of Heart Problems

1. CVD Health Disparities. American Heart Association website. https://www.heart.org/idc/groups/heart-public/@wcm/@hcm/@ml/documents/downloadable/ucm_429240.pdf. Accessed August 28, 2016.

2. Caffeine: How much is too much? Mayo Clinic website. http://www.mayoclinic.org/healthy-lifestyle/nutrition-and-healthy-eating/in-depth/caffeine/art-20045678. Updated April 14, 2014. Accessed August 28, 2016.

3. Frequently Asked Questions. Centers for Disease Control Website. http://www.cdc.gov/alcohol/faqs.htm. Updated August 2, 2016. Accessed August 28, 2016.

Chapter 5: Diagnosing Heart Problems

1. Stethoscope. Science Museum's History of Medicine website. http://www.sciencemuseum.org.uk/broughttolife/techniques/stethoscope. Accessed September 6, 2016.

Chapter 7: Circulation Problems and Symptoms

1. Coronary Artery Disease. Texas Heart Institute Website. http://www.texasheart.org/HIC/Topics/Cond/CoronaryArteryDisease.cfm. Updated August 2016. Accessed September 19, 2016.
2. Go AS, Mozaffarian D, Roger VL, et al. Heart Disease and Stroke Statistics—2013 Update: a report from the American Heart Association. Circulation. 2013;127:e6–245. doi:10.1161/CIR.0b013e31828124ad.

Chapter 9: Diagnosing Circulation Problems

1. Antman EM, Anbe DT, Armstrong PW, et al. ACC/AHA Guidelines for the Management of Patients With ST-Elevation Myocardial Infarction—Executive Summary. Circulation. 2004 August 3;110(5):588-636. doi:10.1161/01.CIR.0000134791.68010.FA.

Chapter 11: Treating Heart Attack Patients

1. Coronary Angioplasty: Treatment for Heart Disease. The Society for Cardiovascular Angiography and Interventions website. http://www.secondscount.org/heart-condition-centers/info-detail-2/coronary-angioplasty-treatment-heart-disease-2#.V-ADc_ArI2x. Updated November 11, 2014. Accessed September 19, 2016.
2. Werner Forssmann – Biographical. Nobel Prize website. http://www.nobelprize.org/nobel_prizes/medicine/laureates/1956/forssmann-bio.html. Published 2014. Accessed September 19, 2016.
3. Butala N, Yeh RW. Is Door-to-Balloon Time a Misleading Metric?. American College of Cardiology website. https://www.acc.org/latest-in-cardiology/

articles/2015/06/03/13/23/is-door-to-balloon-time-a-misleading-metric. Published June 4, 2015. Accessed September 19, 2016.

Chapter 12: Circulation Lifestyle Tips

1. 2015 – 2020 Dietary Guidelines for Americans. 8th Edition. Office of Disease Prevention and Health Promotion website. https://health.gov/dietaryguidelines/2015/. Published December 2015. Accessed August 28, 2016.

2. A Report of the Surgeon General: How Tobacco Smoke Causes Disease. Center for Disease Control and Prevention website. http://www.cdc.gov/tobacco/data_statistics/sgr/2010/consumer_booklet/pdfs/consumer.pdf. Published 2010. Accessed August 28, 2016.

3. Physical Activity. President's Council on Fitness, Sports & Nutrition website. http://www.fitness.gov/resource-center/facts-and-statistics/. Accessed September 20, 2016.

Chapter 13: How Your Myocardium Works

1. Our Top 10 Interesting Heart Facts. Heart Health Institute website. http://www.hearthealthinstitute.net/posts-education/our-top-10-interesting-heart-facts/. Updated January 7, 2015. Accessed September 7, 2016.

Chapter 14: Myocardium Problems and Causes

1. Julian D. The forgotten past: The practice of cardiology in the 1950s and now. Eur Heart J. 2000 Aug;21(16):1277-80. doi:10.1053/euhj.2000.2225.

2. O'Keefe JH, Bhatti SK, Bajwa A, DiNicolantonio JJ, Lavie CJ. Alcohol and Cardiovascular Health: The Dose Makes the Poison…or the Remedy. Mayo Clin Proc. 2014 Mar;89(3):382-93. doi:10.1016/j.mayocp.2013.11.005.

3. Avraham R. *The Circulatory System.* Philadelphia, PA: Chelsea House Publishers; 2000.

Chapter 16: Treating Myocardium Problems

1. Azad N, Lemay G. Management of chronic heart failure in the older population. J Geriatr Cardiol. 2014 Dec; 11(4):329–337. doi:10.11909/j.issn.1671-5411.2014.04.008.

2. Robert Jarvik, MD on the Jarvik-7. Jarvik Heart website. http://www.jarvikheart.com/history/robert-jarvik-on-the-jarvik-7/. Updated 2016. Accessed September 26, 2016.

Chapter 17: Myocardium Lifestyle Tips

1. Processed Foods: Where is all that salt coming from? American Heart Association website. http://www.heart.org/HEARTORG/Healthy-Living/HealthyEating/Nutrition/Processed-Foods-Where-is-all-that-salt-coming-from_UCM_426950_Article.jsp#.V9d46JgrI2w. Updated April 2014. Accessed August 28, 2016.

Chapter 19: Rhythm Problems

1. What is Atrial Fibrillation (AFib or AF)?. American Heart Association website. http://www.heart.org/HEARTORG/Conditions/Arrhythmia/AboutArrhythmia/What-is-Atrial-Fibrillation-AFib-or-AF_UCM_423748_Article.jsp#.V9oTg5grI2x. Updated September 2, 2016. Accessed September 14, 2016.

Chapter 21: Diagnosing and Monitoring Rhythm Problems

1. Patel AY; Eagle KA, Vaishnava P. Cardiac Risk of Noncardiac Surgery. J Am Coll Cardiol.2015;66(19):2140-48.doi:10.1016/j.jacc.2015.09.026.

2. Patel AY; Eagle KA, Vaishnava P. Cardiac Risk of Noncardiac Surgery. J Am Coll Cardiol.2015;66(19):2140-48.doi:10.1016/j.jacc.2015.09.026.

3. Bonner, Robin C. *The Heart and Circulatory System.* Pleasantville, NY: The Reader's Digest Association, Inc.: 2000.

Chapter 23: Rhythm Lifestyle Tips

1. Kodama S, Saito K, Tanaka S, et al. Alcohol consumption and risk of atrial fibrillation: a meta-analysis. J Am Coll Cardiol. 2011 Jan 25;57(4):427-36. doi:10.1016/j.jacc.2010.08.641.

2. Shin J, Roughead EE, Park B, Pratt NL. Cardiovascular safety of methylphenidate among children and young people with attention-deficit/hyperactivity disorder (ADHD): nationwide self controlled case series study. BMJ. 2016;353:i3123. doi:http://dx.doi.org/10.1136/bmj.i2550.

3. Ghuran A, Nolan J. The cardiac complications of recreational drug use. J Med. 2000 Dec; 173(6): 412–415. doi:10.1136/ewjm.173.6.412.

Chapter 24: How Your Valves Work

1. 22 Amazing Facts About Your Heart (Infographic). Cleveland Clinic website. https://health.clevelandclinic.org/2016/08/22-amazing-facts-about-your-heart-infographic/. Updated August 2, 2016. Accessed September 6, 2016.

2. Fedak, PWM, Verma, S, David TE, Leask RL, Weisel RD, Butany J. Clinical and Pathophysiological Implications of a Bicuspid Aortic Valve. Circulation. 2002;106(8) 900-04. doi:10.1136/bmj.i2874.

Chapter 26: Causes of Valve Problems

1. Julian D. The forgotten past: The practice of cardiology in the 1950s and now. Eur Heart J. 2000 Aug;21(16):1277-80. doi:10.1053/euhj.2000.2225.

Chapter 28: Treating Valve Problems

1. Lampropulos JF, Bikdeli B, Gupta A, et al. Most Important Outcomes Research Papers on Valvular Heart Disease. Circulation: Cardiovascular

Quality and Outcomes. 2012;5:e95-e103 doi:10.1161/CIRCOUT-COMES.112.969766.

2. Lampropulos JF, Bikdeli B, Gupta A, et al. Most Important Outcomes Research Papers on Valvular Heart Disease. Circulation: Cardiovascular Quality and Outcomes. 2012;5:e95-e103 doi:10.1161/CIRCOUT-COMES.112.969766.

Chapter 29: Valves Lifestyle Tips

1. Infective Endocarditis. American Heart Association website. http://www.heart.org/HEARTORG/Conditions/CongenitalHeartDefects/TheImpactofCongenitalHeartDefects/Infective-Endocarditis_UCM_307108_Article.jsp. Updated February 11, 2016. Accessed August 23, 2016.

Chapter 31: Problems with the Pericardium

1. Khandaker MH, Espinosa RE, Nishimura RA, et al. Pericardial disease: diagnosis and management. Mayo Clin Proc. 2010;85:572–593. http://dx.doi.org/10.4065/mcp.2010.0046.

2. Lily, LS. Treatment of Acute and Recurrent Idiopathic Pericarditis. Circulation.2013;127(16):1723-26.doi:10.1161/CIRCULATIONAHA.111.066365.

3. Our Top 10 Interesting Heart Facts. Heart Health Institute website. http://www.hearthealthinstitute.net/posts-education/our-top-10-interesting-heart-facts/. Updated January 7, 2015. Accessed September 7, 2016.

Chapter 33: Pericardium Lifestyle Tips

1. How the Fight-or-Flight response explains stress. Psychologist World website. https://www.psychologistworld.com/stress/fightflight.php. Accessed August 28, 2016.

2. 1 in 3 adults don't get enough sleep. Center for Disease Control Website. http://www.cdc.gov/media/releases/2016/p0215-enough-sleep.html. Published February 16, 2016. Accessed August 28, 2016.

3. Sleep and Cardiovascular Disease. SecondsCount website. http://www.secondscount.org/healthy-living/healthy-living-detail?cid=828f98c1-fcb1-4e03-8af3-2e433847be3f#.V8OSZWXdTFI. Accessed August 28, 2016.

Chapter 35: Aorta Problems and Symptoms

1. Tsiaras A. *The InVision Guide to a Healthy Heart.* New York, NY: HarperCollins Publishers; 2005.

Chapter 36: Causes of Aorta Problems

1. Abdominal aortic aneurysm. Mayo Clinic website. http://www.mayoclinic.org/diseases-conditions/abdominal-aortic-aneurysm/symptoms-causes/dxc-20197861. Updated March 23, 2016. Accessed September 1, 2016.

2. Aortic Aneurysm – Cause. Center for Disease Control Website. http://www.cdc.gov/dhdsp/data_statistics/fact_sheets/docs/fs_aortic_aneurysm.pdf. Updated September 9, 2016. Accessed September 1, 2016.

Chapter 37: Diagnosing Aorta Problems

1. Abdominal Aortic Aneurysm: Screening. U.S. Preventative Services Task Force website. http://www.uspreventiveservicestaskforce.org/Page/Document/RecommendationStatementFinal/abdominal-aortic-aneurysm-screening. Published June 2014. Accessed September 1, 2016.

2. Bhattacharyya. R. Top 10 Famous People with Marfan Syndrome. Listovative website. http://listovative.com/top-10-famous-people-with-marfan-syndrome/. Updated 2014. Accessed September 27, 2016.

Chapter 38: Treating Aorta Problems

1. Aortic Dissection - Topic Overview. WebMD website. http://www.webmd.com/heart-disease/tc/aortic-dissection-topic-overview?page=3. Updated September 9, 2014. Accessed September 1, 2016.

Chapter 39: Aorta Lifestyle Tips

1. Donovan J. How Fiber Protects Your Heart. WebMD website. http://www.webmd.com/diet/features/fiber-heart. Updated July 22, 2015. Accessed August 28, 2016.
2. Dietary Fiber. Mayo Clinic website. http://www.mayoclinic.org/healthy-lifestyle/nutrition-and-healthy-eating/in-depth/fiber/art-20043983?pg=2). Updated September 22, 2015. Accessed September 7, 2016.

Glossary

A

Abdominal aorta, section of aorta from the abdomen down

Abdominal aortic aneurysm (AAA), an outward bulge in the wall of the aorta from the abdomen down

Ablation, destruction/deactivation of tissue creating a malfunction

ACE inhibitor, a drug used for the treatment of hypertension and congestive heart failure

Acute coronary syndrome (ACS), an umbrella term for a range of conditions in which blood flow to the heart is suddenly blocked or reduced; commonly called a heart attack

Acute heart failure, sudden onset of heart failure

Adenosine stress test, see pharmacological stress test

Aldosterone antagonists, medicines that help the body get rid of extra water

Angina, severe pain caused by inadequate blood supply to the heart

Angiogram (invasive angiography), a test that uses dye and X-rays to show the insides of your coronary arteries

Angioplasty, procedure used to temporarily widen an artery

Angiotensin-converting enzyme inhibitor, see ACE inhibitor

Anti-arrhythmic drugs (AAD), medications that work to suppress rapid heartbeats by manipulating the heart's electricity

Anticoagulants, blood thinners that reduce the formation of fibrin

Antiplatelets, blood thinners that prevent platelets from bonding together

Antithrombotics, blood thinners

Aorta, artery extending from the heart's left ventricle through which blood flows to the rest of the body

Aortic aneurysm, an outward bulge in the aortic wall

Aortic arch, curved section above the ascending aorta

Aortic dissection, condition that occurs when a tear forms in the innermost layer of the aortic wall and blood leaks through

Aortic valve, valve leading out of the left ventricle

Arrhythmia, a problem with the rate or rhythm of the heartbeat

Arteriosclerosis, buildup of plaque inside blood vessel walls

Ascending aorta, the two inch section of aorta that reaches upward from the heart

Atherosclerosis, hardening of the arteries caused by plaque buildup

Atrial fibrillation or flutter (Afib), a problem with the electrical fibers in the atria

Atrioventricular (AV) node, part of the heart's electrical system

Atrium, a chamber through which blood enters the heart; divided into right and left, the atria comprise the top floors of the heart

AV blockers (av-nodal blockers), drugs that help suppress the junction box or AV node, thus slowing a patient's short circuits or arrhythmias; they can suppress all 6 parts of the electrical system

AVN block, a partial or complete interruption of the heart's electrical signal between the atria and the ventricles

AVN nodal tachycardia (AVNRT), a problem with the AV node

B

Bacterial endocarditis, an infection of the inner lining of the heart muscle and heart valves

Beta blockers, medications that decrease the heart rate by reducing the electrical impulses sent through the AV node

Bicuspid aortic valve disease, a congenital defect of the aortic valve experienced by 1 to 2% of the population

Bioprosthesis, an artificial heart valve containing animal tissue

Biventricular pacemaker, implantable device that helps the left ventricle contract

Bradycardia, an abnormally slow heartbeat

Broken heart syndrome, see Takotsubo cardiomyopathy

Bundle branch block, a condition in which there is a delay along the pathway that electrical impulses travel to make the heart beat

Bundle of His, part of the heart's electrical system

C

CAD, see coronary artery disease

Calcification, accumulation of calcium in the walls of the coronary arteries

Calcium channel blockers, like beta blockers, these drugs decrease the heart rate by reducing the electrical impulses sent through the AV node

Calcium score, a measurement of calcification of the arteries

Cardiac arrest, the abrupt cessation of a heartbeat

Cardiac biomarker, enzymes in the blood that can be used to measure and assess the degree and type of heart damage following a heart attack

Cardiac catheterization, a medical procedure used to diagnose and treat heart conditions; a long, thin, flexible tube is passed into a blood vessel in the arm, groin, or neck and threaded to the heart, where it can be used for diagnostic tests and treatment

Cardiac CT scan, detects calcium buildup and plaque in artery walls and abnormalities in the heart

Cardiac electrophysiologist, diagnoses and treats heart rhythm abnormalities

Cardiac imaging specialist, medical professional who performs and interprets cardiac imaging studies

Cardiac output, the volume of blood your heart pumps in one minute

Cardiac resynchronization therapy device (CRT), a mechanism that coordinates contractions between the left and right ventricles

Cardiac veins, blood vessels that carry blood from the myocardium to the right atrium

Cardiomyopathy, heart muscle disease

Cardiothoracic surgeon, medical professional who performs surgical procedures related to the heart

Cardiovascular surgeon, see cardiothoracic surgeon

Cardiovascular system, the heart and blood vessels that circulate blood and oxygen around the body

Cardioversion, brief electrical shock to the heart through the chest wall designed to disrupt the heart's abnormal electrical circuit and reset it to a normal rhythm

Cardioverter-defibrillator, a small device placed in the chest or abdomen to treat arrhythmias

Catecholamines, hormones made by your adrenal glands as a reaction to stress

Catheter ablation, procedure that involves threading a catheter through an artery in the patient's arm or leg to reduce Afib

Catheter, a long, thin, flexible tube

Catheterization laboratory, room staffed with specialists that is reserved for performing percutaneous coronary intervention; also called a cath lab

Chest X-ray, creates pictures of the structures inside the chest using electromagnetic waves

CHF, see congestive heart failure

Cholesterol, a waxy, fat-like substance found in all cells of the body, including blood cells

Chronic constrictive pericarditis, scarring and damage to the heart muscle caused by an ongoing inflammation

Chronic obstructive pulmonary disease, an umbrella term for diseases of the lungs including asthma, chronic bronchitis, and emphysema

Classic angina, see stable angina

Colchicine, an anti-inflammatory originally used to prevent pericarditis from returning

Computed tomography, an advanced imaging system that can take detailed pictures of your heart

Computerized tomography coronary angiogram, see computed tomography

Congestive heart failure, a weakness of the heart that leads to a buildup of fluid in the lungs and surrounding body tissues

COPD, see chronic obstructive pulmonary disease

Cor pulmonale, right heart failure

Coronary arteries, left and right blood vessels that carry blood from the aorta to the heart

Coronary artery bypass grafting (CABG), surgery in which a healthy artery or vein is connected to a blocked coronary artery in such a way to carry blood flow around the blocked section

Coronary artery disease, a serious condition caused by buildup of plaque in the arteries

Coronary artery stenosis, plaque buildup leading to the narrowing of arteries and restriction of blood flow

Coronary CT angiogram (CCTA), tool used to assess the coronary arteries and detect blockages

Coronary heart disease, see coronary artery disease

Coronary stent, a metal mesh tube used to expand the artery walls to keep the artery open

C-reactive protein (CRP), substance produced by the liver in response to inflammation that could indicate the presence of heart disease

CT, see computed tomography

Cyanosis, bluish tint caused by lack of oxygen

Cystic medial necrosis, a disease involving cyst-like spaces in the muscle fibers of the aorta

D

Decompensated heart failure, see acute heart failure

Defibrillator, a device that delivers an electrical shock to the heart

Depolarization, tiny electrical changes in the heart, measured by an electrocardiogram, that cause the heart muscle to contract

Descending aorta, section of aorta beneath the arch that reaches downward through the chest

Diabetes, a disease of elevated glucose in the blood caused by an inability to produce sufficient insulin

Diastole, the resting phase of the heart

Diastolic heart failure, the decline in the performance of the heart during the resting phase because one or both heart ventricles become stiff and can't fill effectively

Dilated cardiomyopathy, a condition in which the heart muscle stretches and becomes thinner, leading to heart failure

Diuretics, medications that increase the flow of urine

Dobutamine stress test, see pharmacological stress test

Door-to-balloon, the time between arrival at a hospital and a catheterization procedure

Doppler ultrasound, a diagnostic tool that shows the speed and direction of blood flow through the valves

E

ECG, see electrocardiogram

Echocardiogram, an ultrasound image of the heart

Ejection fraction (EF), a measurement of the amount of blood ejected from the heart with each beat

EKG, see electrocardiogram

Electrocardiogram, a test that measures the electrical impulses of the heart

Electrophysiology (EP), the study of the electrical properties of the body's systems

Endovascular aneurysm repair (EVAR), method of repairing an aneurysm by threading a catheter through the groin and using a stent graft

Epicardium, see visceral pericardium

Event monitor, an electrocardiogram device that monitors the heart's activity over a week or month

Exercise nuclear test, a procedure that enables a doctor to look for heart blockages by injecting radioactive dye into the bloodstream and having the patient walk on a treadmill

Exercise stress test, a procedure that enables a doctor to measure the heart's performance during physical activity

F

Fibrillation, an electrical disorder of the heart

Fibrin, a strong protein that combines with blood platelets to form blood clots

Fibrosis, scarring

H

HCM, see hypertrophic cardiomyopathy

HDL, see high-density lipoprotein cholesterol

Heart attack, a disruption of the flow of oxygenated blood to the muscle of the heart; see acute coronary syndrome or ACS

Heart catheterization, see cardiac catheterization

Heart disease risk factor, condition that can increase a person's chance of developing heart problems; a risk factor can be congenital (present at birth) or acquired (developed over a lifetime)

Heart disease, an umbrella term for a range of conditions affecting your heart

Heart failure, a condition in which the heart can't pump enough blood to meet the body's needs

Heart murmur, see murmur

High blood pressure, a condition in which blood flows through arteries at higher than normal pressures

High-density lipoprotein cholesterol, so-called "good cholesterol"

HMG-CoA reductase inhibitor, see statin

Holiday heart syndrome, arrhythmia in an otherwise healthy person who has ingested large amounts of alcohol over a brief period

Hypertension, see high blood pressure

Hypertensive heart disease, stiffening of the heart muscle caused by high blood pressure

Hypertrophic cardiomyopathy (HCM), genetically induced enlarged and thickened heart muscle

I

Idiopathic, occurring without any known cause

Imaging stress test, provides images showing the blood flow to the heart at rest and during exercise

Implantable cardioverter defibrillator, a device which prevents life-threatening arrhythmias

Implantable loop recorder (ILR), a device implanted under the skin of the chest near the heart used to record the heart's electrical activity on a continuous basis

Innocent heart murmur, a non-threatening heart murmur

Interventional cardiologist, a specialist who diagnoses and treats problems in the blood vessels and cardiovascular system

Intraventricular conduction delay (IVCD), a slowing or block in the ventricular fibers

Ischemia, a restriction of blood supply to an organ or tissue

Ischemic cardiomyopathy, heart wall damage due to lack of oxygen reaching the heart

L

LDL cholesterol, see low-density lipoprotein cholesterol

Left anterior descending artery (LAD), supplies blood to the front of the heart

Left bundle branch (LBB), part of the heart's electrical system

Left circumflex artery (LCX), supplies blood to the back of the heart

Left or right bundle branch block, an interruption of the electrical signal somewhere in the left or right bundle branches of the heart

Left or right bundle branch ventricular tachycardia, a problem or short circuit with the LBB or RBB

Left ventricle hypertrophy, thickening of the left ventricle

Left ventricular dilatation, thinning of the left ventricle

Left ventricular ejection fraction, see ejection fraction (EF)

Low-density lipoprotein cholesterol, so-called "bad" cholesterol

Luminal stenosis, medical term for narrowing of the arteries

Lyme carditis, a complication of Lyme disease

M

Marfan Syndrome, a connective tissue disorder

Mechanical circulatory support, manufactured technology used to assist heart failure patients when other means have proven ineffective

Mechanical valve, a man-made valve used to replace an abnormal heart valve

Mitral valve, valve through which blood from the left atrium flows into the left ventricle

Mobile EKG, a smartphone app that can record and transmit EKG data from a patient to a doctor

MRI, see magnetic resonance imaging

Murmur, an extra or unusual sound heard during a heartbeat

Myectomy, removal of parts of the heart that have become too enlarged, weak, or stiff to function properly in order to improve blood flow and allow the healthy part of the heart to continue pumping

Myocardial infarction, see heart attack

Myocardial ischemia, a lack of oxygen to the heart due to narrowed arteries

Myocarditis, damage caused by infections in the heart

Myocardium, the muscular wall of the heart

N

Nitrates, drugs that dilate the arteries to the heart, improving blood flow

Noninvasive, not involving puncturing the skin or entering the body

Non-ischemic cardiomyopathy, heart damage caused by issues other than restricted blood and oxygen flow

Non-obstructive coronary artery disease, less than a 70% reduction of blood flow to the heart caused by stable plaque buildup in the arteries

NSTEMI, a heart attack resulting from a blocked artery that has caused cell death

Nuclear stress test, a stress test in which a radioactive substance is injected into the bloodstream, enabling the heart to be imaged both at rest and under stress

O

Obstructive coronary artery disease, a 70% or greater reduction of blood flow to the heart caused by plaque buildup and narrowing of the arteries

Obstructive sleep apnea (OSA), pauses in breathing during sleep indicating partial obstruction of the upper airway caused by excess body tissue (e.g. fat)

P

Pacemaker, an implanted mechanical device that regulates the rhythm of the heart

Parietal pericardium, the outer layer of the pericardium that anchors the heart in place

PCI, see percutaneous coronary intervention

Percutaneous coronary intervention, methods used to restore blood flow in the heart, such as angioplasty with stenting and bypass surgery

Pericardial effusion, an abnormal accumulation of fluid around the heart

Pericardial sac, acts as a cushion for the heart

Pericardial stripping, ultrasound-guided procedure that drains the excess fluid from the pericardial sac using a large needle

Pericardial window, a surgical incision made to drain fluid from the pericardium

Pericardiocentesis, an ultrasound-guided procedure that drains the excess fluid from the pericardial sac using a large needle

Pericarditis, inflammation of the pericardium

Pericardium, the membrane that surrounds the heart

Peripheral arteries, vessels that carry blood to the head, organs, and limbs

Pharmacological stress test, a stress test that uses medication in place of physical exercise

Plaque, buildup of excess fat, cholesterol, calcium, and other substances found in the blood

Platelets, blood cell fragments that, combined with fibrin, can keep a blood clot from breaking apart

Pleural effusion, excess fluid around the lungs

Pulmonary artery, vessel that carries oxygen-depleted blood from the heart to the lungs

Pulmonary edema, fluid in the lungs

Pulmonary hypertension, increased pressure in the pulmonary arteries

Pulmonary valve, valve between the right ventricle and the pulmonary artery

Pulmonary veins, vessels that carry oxygenated blood from the lungs to the heart

Purkinje (ventricular) fibers, part of the heart's electrical system

Purkinje ventricular tachycardia, a problem of the ventricles' electrical fibers

R

Regurgitation, backflow or leaking of blood back into the chambers that occurs if a valve doesn't close tightly

Reverse remodeling, a process during which an unhealthy heart wall begins to heal, allowing it to function in a healthier fashion

Rheumatic fever, a consequence of untreated strep infection which can cause heart valve damage

Right bundle branch (RBB), part of the heart's electrical system

S

Sinoatrial (SA) node, part of the heart's electrical system that starts the heartbeat

Sinus bradycardia, a problem with the sinus node

Sinus node, the natural pacemaker of the heart

Sinus rhythm, the natural rhythm of the heart

Sinus tachycardia, a problem with the sinus node

Sleep apnea, pauses in breathing during sleep

Sonography, see ultrasound

Stable angina, predictable chest pain caused by activity and stress

Stable plaque, calcium-rich buildup in the arteries that is less likely to rupture

Statin, a common medication that helps reduce bad cholesterol

STEMI, a heart attack resulting from a complete and prolonged blockage of an artery in the heart

Stenosis, an abnormal narrowing of a passage in the body

Stenotic valve, a valve with thickened, stiffened or fused leaflets

Stent, a small mesh tube used to treat narrow or weak arteries

Stethoscope, medical device used to listen to the heart and other sounds in the body

Stress test, a diagnostic test measuring heart function both at rest and during exercise

Stroke, a disruption of the supply of oxygenated blood to the brain

Sudden cardiac death, a condition in which the heart suddenly and unexpectedly stops beating

Supraventricular tachycardia, a fast heart rate that begins in the upper chamber of the heart

Syncope, fainting

Systole, the contraction phase of the heart

Systolic CHF, see systolic congestive heart failure

Systolic congestive heart failure, a condition in which the heart walls contract only partially and expel only a fraction of the blood they normally send out into the body

T

Tachy-brady syndrome, a condition in which the heart sometimes beats too slowly and other times too quickly

Tachycardia, an abnormally rapid heartbeat

Takotsubo cardiomyopathy, the abrupt onset of symptoms related to wall damage which occurs during or directly after high levels of stress

Tamponade, compression of the heart caused by fluid buildup

Tertiary care hospital, specialized care hospital

Thoracic aorta, section of aorta above the diaphragm

Thoracic aortic aneurysm (TAA), a bulge in the section of aortic wall above the diaphragm

Thromboembolism, obstruction of blood flow caused by a clot

Thrombolytics, clot buster medications

Thrombosis, formation of a blood clot that blocks an artery

Thrombus, medical term for blood clot

Tilt-table test, special table used to determine if there's an association between the patient's body position and symptoms

Transcatheter aortic valve replacement (TAVR), means of repairing the aortic valve by threading a catheter through an artery

Transesophageal echocardiography (TEE), a transducer attached to the end of a flexible tube, which is then guided down the throat and into the esophagus in order to view the heart

Transient ischemic attack (TIA), a mini-stroke

Treadmill stress test, see exercise stress test

Tricuspid valve, valve between the right atrium and right ventricle

Triglycerides, type of fat in the blood linked to heart disease

Troponin, a protein that helps muscles contract, detectable in the blood when heart muscle is damaged

U

Ultrasound, high-frequency sound waves that produce pictures of the heart

Unstable angina, unpredictable chest pain that comes on suddenly

Unstable plaque, lipid-rich buildup in the arteries that is likely to rupture

V

Valve endocarditis, an infection in the valves of the heart

Valve-induced cardiomyopathy, weakening of the heart caused by stenotic valves

Valves, flaps that allow blood to flow from one chamber to another

Valvular heart disease, an illness caused by a poorly functioning valve

Vasovagal response (vasovagal syncope), a drop in heart rate and blood pressure that results in lightheadedness, faded vision and loss of consciousness

Vena cava, the two large veins through which oxygen-depleted blood enters into the heart from other parts of the body; called the superior vena cava and the inferior vena cava

Ventricle, a chamber through which blood leaves the heart; divided into right and left, the ventricles comprise the bottom floor of the heart

Ventricular assist device (VAD), a mechanical pump used to support heart function and blood flow in patients with weakened hearts

Ventricular fibrillation (Vfib), a life-threatening disturbance in the heart's rhythm that prevents the heart from pumping blood properly, leading to cardiac arrest

Ventricular tachycardia, a fast rhythm that starts in the heart's lower chambers

Viral myocarditis, heart inflammation caused by a virus

Visceral pericardium, comprised of two inner layers of the pericardium: one that surrounds the heart and another that is attached to the outer layer

Vulnerable plaque, see stable plaque

Index